KETO DIET BOOK FOR BEGINNERS OVER 60

A Comprehensive Journey to Wellness with Delicious Recipes, Nutrient Insights, and a Meal Plan – Revitalize Your Health, Reverse the Clock, and Regain Your Life!

Linda Hudson

TABLE OF CONTENTS

INTRODUCTION

Welcome, dear reader, to a transformative journey that has the potential to reshape not just your diet but your overall health and vitality. As a seasoned nutritional specialist with a wealth of experience guiding individuals toward healthier lifestyles, I am thrilled to introduce you to the world of the ketogenic diet. This lifestyle choice has proven particularly beneficial for those in their golden years.

You might be wondering, "Is the keto diet right for me at this stage of life?". The answer is a resounding yes! The keto diet, a science-backed approach to eating, can help regulate blood sugar, improve mental clarity, boost energy levels, and even assist in weight management. These benefits are especially crucial for maintaining health as we age, making the keto diet an ideal choice for you.

In this book, I've tailored the keto diet specifically for beginners over 60, considering this age group's unique nutritional needs and health considerations. You'll find a comprehensive guide to understanding the keto diet basics, including the science of ketosis, how to balance macronutrients, and how to read nutrition labels effectively. But it's not just about theory. I've also included practical tips, from setting up your keto-friendly kitchen to navigating dining out. And, of course, the keto guide is only complete with delicious recipes and a detailed meal plan to help you embark on this journey with confidence and ease. So, whether you're looking to manage a health condition, boost your energy levels, or embrace a healthier lifestyle, this book is designed to provide you with the knowledge and tools you need to succeed. Let's embark on this journey together and discover the many benefits the keto diet offers for your golden years.

Welcome to the Keto Journey: A Beginner's Guide for Older People

As a nutritional specialist, I am thrilled to welcome you to the start of your keto journey. The ketogenic diet, with its focus on healthy fats and low carbohydrates, offers a pathway to better health that is particularly well-suited to the needs of older individuals.

Embracing the keto lifestyle can be a transformative experience. It's about more than just changing your diet; it's about adopting a new approach to eating that can help you manage your weight, enhance your mental clarity, and boost your energy levels. These benefits are precious as we age and face unique health challenges.

Starting a new diet can be daunting, but I'm here to guide you. The key to success is understanding which foods to include, such as leafy greens, avocados, olive oil, fish, and chicken, and which to avoid, like sugary snacks and high-carb bread. It's also important to stay hydrated and get enough electrolytes, especially during the initial adjustment period.

Remember, this journey is about finding what works best for you. Listen to your body, make adjustments as needed, and seek support from healthcare professionals or fellow keto enthusiasts.

Understanding the Keto Diet: Basics and Benefits

The ketogenic diet is more than just a trend; it's a lifestyle many have embraced for its numerous health benefits. The keto diet is about shifting your body's primary fuel source from carbohydrates to fats. This metabolic state, ketosis, is achieved by significantly reducing carb intake and increasing healthy fat consumption.

But what makes the keto diet particularly beneficial? It can improve weight management by encouraging the body to burn fat for energy. Additionally, many people on the keto diet report increased mental clarity and focus and more stable energy levels throughout the day.

These benefits can be especially impactful for seniors. Managing weight becomes more challenging with age, and cognitive health is a priority for maintaining independence and quality of life. By adopting a keto lifestyle, you're not just changing your diet; you're investing in your long-term health and well-being.

The keto diet also supports heart health by promoting reduced triglyceride levels and increased HDL (good) cholesterol. This can be particularly beneficial for older adults who are at a higher risk for cardiovascular diseases.

As you delve deeper into the keto diet, you'll discover a world of delicious, nutritious foods that support your health goals. Embrace the journey and enjoy the benefits of this transformative way of eating

Why Keto is Especially Beneficial for Older Adults

The golden years bring many joys but can also present unique health challenges. As a nutritional specialist, I've seen firsthand how the ketogenic diet can offer specific advantages for older adults looking to maintain their health and vitality.

One of the most significant benefits is the potential for improved metabolic health. With age, the risk of conditions like type 2 diabetes and metabolic syndrome increases. By reducing carbohydrate intake and stabilizing blood sugar levels, the keto diet can be an effective tool in managing these risks.

Furthermore, the keto diet's emphasis on healthy fats and quality proteins can support muscle maintenance and bone health—both critical for mobility and independence in later life. The anti-inflammatory properties of many keto-friendly foods can also help reduce chronic pain and improve joint health.

Lastly, the cognitive benefits of the keto diet should be noticed. Research suggests that a low-carb, high-fat diet can support brain health and may even offer protective benefits against conditions like Alzheimer's disease.

In addition to these benefits, the keto diet can aid digestion and gut health, which can be particularly important for seniors who may experience digestive issues. The high fiber content in keto-friendly vegetables can promote a healthy gut microbiome. Incorporating the keto diet into your lifestyle as an older adult can be a proactive step towards preserving your health and enjoying your years to the fullest. It's always possible to start making positive changes for your well-being.

CHAPTER 1:
COMPREHENSIVE HEALTH
CONSIDERATIONS FOR SENIORS OVER 60

Maintaining health and wellness becomes increasingly important for seniors over 60. A well-planned ketogenic diet can be tailored to meet the unique nutritional requirements and health challenges that arise during this time for both men and women. This chapter will discuss the keto diet's role in addressing these concerns, ensuring a holistic approach to senior health.

Hormonal Changes and Keto: Managing Menopause and Andropause Symptoms

Navigating Hormonal Shifts with Keto

The hormonal changes experienced during menopause and andropause can be significant. Women may contend with hot flashes and mood swings, while men might face decreased libido and energy levels. The ketogenic diet has been associated with improved insulin sensitivity, which might influence other hormones, potentially easing these symptoms.

For women, incorporating phytoestrogens, and for men, focusing on zinc and fatty acids for testosterone support can be advantageous. Tailoring the diet to include foods like flaxseeds for women and oysters for men, along with maintaining a balanced keto diet, can aid in managing the hormonal fluctuations associated with age.

Bone Density and Osteoporosis: Keto and Calcium Intake for Seniors

Keto's Role in Protecting Senior Bone Health

Calcium's role in maintaining bone health is well-documented, and the risk of osteoporosis is a significant concern for seniors. A ketogenic diet rich in calcium from leafy greens, cheese, and almonds, paired with vitamin D and magnesium, can support bone density.

After consulting healthcare providers, seniors should aim for calcium-rich keto-friendly options and consider supplements. Regular weight-bearing exercises like walking and resistance training will complement dietary efforts to strengthen bones.

Heart Health: Reducing Risk Factors for Cardiovascular Disease in Seniors

The Ketogenic Diet and Senior Cardiovascular Wellness

The ketogenic diet can support heart health by positively affecting blood pressure, cholesterol levels, and weight management—critical cardiovascular risk factors. Incorporating omega-3s and avoiding trans fats is vital for seniors pursuing a heart-healthy keto lifestyle.

Monitoring the types of fats consumed and ensuring a variety of fatty acids, particularly those from fish, nuts, and seeds, is essential. Regular cardiovascular check-ups will help tailor the diet to individual health profiles.

Prostate and Breast Cancer Prevention: Diet and Lifestyle Factors for Seniors

Keto and Cancer Prevention in the Senior Years

The correlation between diet and cancer is an area of active research. For seniors, a ketogenic diet may contribute to lowering the risk factors associated with prostate and breast cancer by reducing insulin levels and inflammation.

Foods high in antioxidants, selenium, lycopene, and sulforaphane support overall health and may have specific prostate and breast health benefits. For cancer risk management, a focus on whole, unprocessed foods within the ketogenic framework is recommended.

Muscle Maintenance and Sarcopenia Prevention in Older Men

Maintaining Muscle Mass with Keto After 60

Preserving muscle mass with advancing age is crucial to maintaining mobility and overall health. Sarcopenia, the age-related loss of muscle mass and strength, mainly affects older men. A ketogenic diet with adequate amounts of high-quality protein can support muscle health.

Eating enough protein from lean meats, fish, and plant-based options like tempeh and combining this with resistance training exercises can be particularly effective against sarcopenia. Seniors should adjust their protein intake based on their activity level and health needs in consultation with health professionals.

Cognitive Function and Keto: Brain Health in Seniors

Supporting Cognitive Health with Keto

Maintaining cognitive function becomes a critical health concern as we enter our senior years. The ketogenic diet has been studied for its potential benefits in brain health, possibly due to its ability to provide a steady source of energy in ketones, which can be particularly beneficial for aging brains.

Incorporating foods rich in omega-3 fatty acids, antioxidants, and B vitamins within a ketogenic framework can support cognitive function. Regular mental exercises and social engagement are lifestyle factors that work in tandem with diet to promote cognitive health.

This comprehensive approach to keto for seniors over 60 aims to address the various health aspects that aging impacts. It's essential to tailor dietary choices to individual health concerns and lifestyle preferences, constantly in alignment with guidance from healthcare providers.

Sexual Health and Keto: Considerations for Seniors

Enhancing Sexual Well-being with a Ketogenic Lifestyle

Sexual health is an essential aspect of life quality, which can also be affected by nutritional choices in the senior years. For many, a ketogenic diet can improve circulation and energy levels, potentially enhancing sexual health. It's also essential for seniors to include foods that support vascular health and hormone balance, such as fatty fish, nuts, avocados, and olive oil, which provide essential fats that are critical components in hormone production.

Careful attention to cardiovascular health through the keto diet may improve sexual health by improving heart function and blood flow. Of course, any concerns in this area should be openly discussed with a healthcare provider, as they can provide personalized advice and support.

Mental Health and Emotional Well-being on Keto

Keto's Impact on Mental and Emotional Health for Seniors

Mental and emotional well-being is as important as physical health, especially for seniors. The ketogenic diet has been associated with mood stabilization, which could be beneficial for those experiencing the emotional fluctuations that can come with aging.

A diet rich in omega-3 fatty acids, abundant in a ketogenic diet, supports mental health. Additionally, the structured nature of the diet and the focus on nourishment can give seniors a sense of control and accomplishment, positively impacting their mental health. Pairing this with regular social interaction and activities that promote mental clarity and emotional balance is vital for holistic well-being.

By approaching the ketogenic diet with a focus on comprehensive health for seniors over 60, including both men and women, we can support longevity and quality of life. Every individual's journey is unique, and dietary plans should be adjusted to meet personal health histories and goals, always in consultation with health professionals.

CHAPTER 2:
KETO BASICS FOR BEGINNERS

As a nutritional specialist, it's my pleasure to welcome you to a path that weaves through history and health—a path known as the ketogenic diet. This chapter is not just an introduction to a diet; it's an invitation to be part of a legacy that has nurtured well-being for almost a century. Before diving into the keto diet, let's begin with the History of the Ketogenic Diet.

The Historical Tapestry of the Ketogenic Diet

The ketogenic diet, now embraced for its health and wellness benefits, has a tapestry rich with historical and medicinal threads. Its origins date back to the early 20th century when it first emerged not for weight loss or metabolic syndrome but as a therapeutic diet to treat epilepsy.

In the 1920s, Dr. Russell Wilder at the Mayo Clinic coined the term "ketogenic diet" and formalized its use for managing epilepsy in children. The diet mimicked the biochemical changes of fasting, which had long been recognized for its seizure-controlling properties, by inducing a state of ketosis through a high-fat, low-carbohydrate diet. Remarkably, for many patients, the frequency and intensity of seizures were significantly reduced without the need for fasting.

Through the mid-century, the advent of anticonvulsant medications led to the diet's decline. However, a resurgence of interest occurred in the 1990s, sparked by the story of Charlie Abrahams, the son of Hollywood producer

Jim Abrahams. The ketogenic diet successfully managed Charlie's severe epilepsy after medications failed. Inspired by his son's dramatic improvement, Jim Abrahams founded the Charlie Foundation to promote the diet and fund research, leading to a renewed scientific interest and a broader diet application beyond epilepsy.

Since then, the ketogenic diet has been explored for various health benefits, including weight loss, diabetes management, and potential roles in cancer therapy, Alzheimer's disease, and other neurological conditions. It has evolved with variations like the Modified Atkins Diet and the Low Glycemic Index Treatment, offering diverse approaches to inducing ketosis.

For seniors today, the history of the ketogenic diet underscores its potential as a powerful tool for health management. Its adaptability and therapeutic roots remind them of the diet's potential to support a range of health goals, from metabolic health to cognitive function.

Embracing the ketogenic diet is to partake in a historical legacy of nutritional healing and well-being. It's a testament to the diet's ability to stand the test of time and science, continually finding new roles in the ever-expanding domain of health and nutrition.

The Science of Ketosis: How It Works in the Aging Body

As we age, our bodies undergo a symphony of changes, and one of the most profound is how we provide energy for our daily activities. The ketogenic diet, rich in history and health benefits, opens the door to ketosis, a metabolic state that can resonate beautifully with the needs of an aging body. Let's explore this elegant science and its implications for seniors.

What is Ketosis?

The body yearns for a symphony of stability in the golden years, and ketosis offers just that. Without sufficient carbohydrates, it's a natural metabolic state where the body turns to fats as its primary energy source. Envision a furnace that once burned wood is now gracefully glowing with a steady, slow-burning coal flame. This is ketosis, a process that transforms fats into ketones, tiny molecules that provide a consistent stream of energy.

For seniors, ketosis is akin to finding an old lamp that, when polished, shines with a renewed light. It's an energy source that can sustain you without the highs and lows of sugar rushes, bringing a new zest to your step and clarity to your mind.

The Role of Insulin in Ketosis

Insulin, the gatekeeper of our cells' glucose uptake, plays a delicate dance with our body's energy levels. As we grow wiser with age, our bodies sometimes struggle to maintain the harmony of this dance. Ketosis introduces a different rhythm, one where insulin takes a gentler path, and our reliance on glucose wanes.

In ketosis, insulin levels typically stabilize due to lower carbohydrate intake. This can be a boon for seniors, as steady insulin levels mean energy levels are less likely to spike or plummet, allowing for a serene energy flow throughout the day.

Benefits of Being in Ketosis

Being in ketosis offers a bouquet of potential benefits, each petal a testament to its power to enhance the lives of seniors. Weight management often becomes a gentle journey rather than a struggle as the body becomes more adept at using stored fat. Cognitive clarity may flourish as ketones prove to be an efficient fuel for the brain, and the stable energy they provide can endow seniors with the endurance to engage fully with each day's joys.

Moreover, ketosis can bring about a sense of peace as the hunger pangs and cravings that once dictated the day's tempo soften, and a satiating calm occurs. For seniors, ketosis isn't just about physical health; it's about cultivating a life where every moment is lived to its fullest, energized by the right foods and a balanced body.

The science of ketosis offers not only a metabolic marvel but also a companion for graceful aging, allowing seniors to embrace the wisdom of their years with vigor and vitality.

Understanding Ketones in the Aging Body

As we journey through the golden years, our bodies seek sources of energy that are both sustaining and gentle. In the ketogenic diet, ketones emerge as a beacon of hope, offering a steady and reliable energy source. Let's delve into ketones, understanding their role and significance in aging.

What are Ketones?

Ketones are the body's ingenious solution to a low-carbohydrate environment. When the intake of carbohydrates is reduced, as in the ketogenic diet, the body's usual energy source, glucose, becomes scarce. In response, the liver initiates a remarkable process, converting fats into ketones, ensuring the body's energy needs are met.

This production of ketones is a testament to the body's adaptability. It's a shift from a glucose-dependent energy system to one that thrives on fats, a change that can bring many benefits, especially for seniors. Ketones provide a smooth and sustained energy flow, unlike the fluctuating energy levels often experienced with glucose. They remind us that even as we age, our bodies can find balance and harmony in new ways.

Types of Ketones and Their Functions

In the intricate dance of our metabolism, ketones play a harmonious trio, each with its unique role in fueling our bodies. Imagine them as three musicians in the orchestra of our energy system, each contributing their melody to the symphony of life.

Acetoacetate is the first ketone produced in the liver from fatty acids. It's like the opening note of a beautiful song, setting the stage for what's to come. Acetoacetate can be considered the pioneer, leading the way for the other ketones to follow.

Beta-Hydroxybutyrate (BHB) is the most abundant and stable ketone. It's the main melody in our symphony, providing the bulk of the energy. BHB is like the steady rhythm that keeps the music flowing, ensuring that every cell can function harmoniously.

Acetone, the least abundant ketone, is produced from the breakdown of acetoacetate. It's like the subtle harmony that adds depth to the song. Although it's not used for energy, the presence of acetone can be an indicator of ketosis, like a gentle whisper telling us that the body is in balance.

For seniors, understanding these types of ketones is like tuning the instruments of their health. Each ketone plays its part in the energy production process, ensuring that the body can continue to perform its functions with grace and vitality. The symphony of ketones is a reminder of the body's remarkable ability to adapt and thrive, even in the golden years.

Measuring Ketone Levels

Measuring ketone levels is like listening to your body's whispers, understanding its rhythm, and ensuring that the melody of ketosis is playing as intended. It's a way of tuning into the harmony of your metabolism, ensuring that your ketogenic journey is on the right path.

There are three primary methods for measuring ketone levels, each with its charm:

- **Blood Ketone Meter:** This method measures the amount of beta-hydroxybutyrate (BHB) in your blood. It's like listening to the heartbeat of your ketosis, providing a precise and real-time snapshot of your metabolic state. A simple finger prick is all it takes to capture this intimate measure of your body's energy source.

- **Breath Ketone Analyzer:** This device measures the amount of acetone in your breath. It's a noninvasive way to detect ketosis, offering a glimpse into how your body is burning fat. Like a gentle breeze carrying the fragrance of a blooming garden, a breath ketone analyzer can reveal the subtle presence of ketones.

- **Urine Ketone Strips:** These strips detect the presence of acetoacetate in your urine. It's quick and easy, like dipping your toes into a stream to gauge its flow. While more precise than blood measurements, urine strips can be a convenient way to get an initial indication of whether you're entering ketosis.

Monitoring ketone levels can be especially important for seniors, as it can help tailor the diet to their unique needs, ensuring smooth energy flow and balanced well-being. It's a way of conducting the orchestra of your health with precision and care, ensuring that every note of your body's symphony is played to perfection.

Macronutrients: Fats, Proteins, and Carbs for Aging Bodies

As we age, the harmony of macronutrients - fats, proteins, and carbohydrates - becomes even more crucial to our well-being. Navigating the golden years with grace and vitality requires understanding how these essential nutrients work together to support our health. Let's explore the art of balancing these macronutrients in a way that nourishes and sustains the aging body.

Balancing Your Macros for Longevity

As we navigate through the golden years, the equilibrium of macronutrients—fats, proteins, and carbohydrates—plays a pivotal role in our overall well-being. This balance is like a beautifully choreographed dance, where each step and movement is essential for maintaining health and vitality.

Fats should take center stage in your meals, providing about 70-75% of your daily caloric intake. They are slow-burning candles that illuminate your days with steady energy. Proteins are the supporting dancers, making up around 20-25% of your intake. They are essential for preserving your strength and independence. Carbohydrates, though limited to 5-10%, are like delicate flourishes that add color and vital nutrients to your diet.

Embracing this balance means you can waltz through your later years with grace, a harmonious blend of nourishment and satisfaction each day.

The Importance of Healthy Fats for Seniors

In the tapestry of a senior's diet, healthy fats are the golden threads that add richness and texture. These fats, such as those found in avocados, olive oil, and nuts, are not just sources of energy; they are the guardians of your heart, the nurturers of your brain, and the soothers of your joints.

Incorporating a variety of healthy fats into your daily meals is like weaving a protective net around your well-being. They help maintain the fluidity of your cell membranes, support cognitive function, and even help keep inflammation at bay. As you savor the creamy texture of an avocado or the rich taste of olive oil, you're not just indulging your taste buds but fortifying your health.

Protein Intake for Muscle Maintenance in Seniors

Protein is the loyal companion that walks with you, hand in hand, through aging. It's the architect that helps maintain the structure and function of your muscles, ensuring that each step you take is as vital as possible.

For seniors, it's crucial to include a variety of protein sources in your diet, such as lean meats, fish, eggs, and legumes. These foods provide the building blocks your body needs to repair tissues and support muscle mass, essential for mobility and independence.

In the golden years, every meal is an opportunity to celebrate the flavors of life while nourishing your body with the essential macronutrients it needs. Embrace the dance of fats, proteins, and carbohydrates, and let them guide you toward a future filled with health and vitality.

In this serene chapter of life, the careful balance of macronutrients becomes the cornerstone of our daily nourishment. Like a skilled gardener tending to a beloved garden, we must tend to our bodies with intention and wisdom, ensuring that each meal is a testament to our commitment to health and vitality.

Fats, the luxurious oils that keep our engines running smoothly, should be chosen with love and care. Embrace the richness of avocados, the wholesomeness of nuts, and the purity of olive oil, each drop promising energy and protection for your heart and mind.

Proteins, the stalwart defenders of our muscle mass, become ever more precious as the years pass. Opt for lean, high-quality sources like fish, chicken, and plant-based. Each bite is a pledge to preserve your strength and independence.

Carbohydrates, though limited, should be selected for their vibrancy and nutrient density. Fill your plate with rainbow colors in the form of leafy greens, berries, and cruciferous vegetables, each mouthful a celebration of life's natural bounty.

In this golden phase, let the art of balancing macronutrients guide you to a life lived with purpose and joy. Each meal is an opportunity to honor the journey you've embarked upon, a chance to nourish not just your body but your soul.

Foods to Enjoy and Avoid: A Beginner's Guide

Embarking on the ketogenic journey is like setting sail on a culinary adventure, where your chosen foods become the anchors of your health and well-being. As we age, this adventure takes on new meaning, with each meal offering an opportunity to nourish our bodies and souls. Let's navigate the waters of keto-friendly foods and those best left ashore, ensuring every bite is a step toward vitality and joy.

Keto-Friendly Foods

Embrace these keto-friendly foods as the cornerstone of your ketogenic journey, each offering its unique blend of nutrients and flavors:

- **Leafy Greens:** Spinach, kale, Swiss chard, arugula
- **Cruciferous Vegetables:** Broccoli, cauliflower, Brussels sprouts, cabbage

- **Fatty Fish:** Salmon, mackerel, sardines, trout
- **Seafood:** Shrimp, crab, lobster, scallops
- **Meats:** Grass-fed beef, pork, lamb, chicken, turkey
- **Eggs:** Free-range or organic eggs
- **Healthy Fats:** Avocados, olive oil, coconut oil, MCT oil
- **Nuts and Seeds:** Almonds, walnuts, chia seeds, flaxseeds, pumpkin seeds
- **Low-Carb Dairy:** Cheese, butter, Greek yogurt, heavy cream
- **Berries:** Strawberries, raspberries, blueberries (in moderation)
- **Herbs and Spices:** Basil, oregano, thyme, cinnamon, turmeric

Foods to Limit or Avoid

While exploring the bounty of keto-friendly foods, be mindful of limiting or avoiding these items to maintain your state of ketosis and support your health goals:

- **Sugary Foods:** Candy, ice cream, cookies, fruit juices, soda
- **Starchy Vegetables:** Potatoes, sweet potatoes, corn, peas, winter squash
- **Grains:** Wheat, rice, oats, barley, quinoa, bread, pasta
- **High-Sugar Fruits:** Bananas, grapes, oranges, apples, mangoes
- **Legumes:** Beans, lentils, chickpeas
- **Processed Foods:** Chips, crackers, cereal bars, processed meats
- **Unhealthy Fats:** Margarine, shortening, vegetable oils (canola, soybean, corn)
- **Alcohol:** Beer, sweet wines, cocktails with high sugar content

Incorporating these lists into your daily meal planning will ensure you're nurturing your body with the right foods, transforming each meal into self-care and a celebration of life's flavors.

Reading Nutrition Labels: What to Look for at Age 60+

The Key to Decoding Nutrition Labels

Understanding nutrition labels becomes an essential skill in the journey of maintaining health and vitality in our senior years. It's like having a compass that guides you through the maze of food choices, ensuring that every turn you take aligns with your nutritional needs and goals. Here's a more detailed guide to the critical components of nutrition labels:

- **Serving Size:** Begin by noting the serving size, as all the nutritional information listed is based on this amount. It's crucial for portion control and understanding how much of each nutrient you consume.

- **Calories:** Check the calories per serving to manage your energy intake. Balancing calorie consumption with your activity level is essential for maintaining a healthy weight.

- **Total Fat:** Look at the total fat content, but also delve deeper into the types of fat present. Opt for foods with higher amounts of healthy fats, such as monounsaturated and polyunsaturated fats, and lower amounts of saturated and trans fats.

- **Cholesterol and Sodium:** While these are necessary in moderation, excessive intake can lead to health issues such as heart disease and high blood pressure. Keep an eye on these, especially if you have specific dietary restrictions.

- **Total Carbohydrates:** This is a critical section for those on a ketogenic diet. Pay attention to the total carbs and the fiber content to calculate net carbs (total carbs minus fiber), which should be kept low to maintain ketosis.

- **Protein:** Protein is vital for muscle maintenance and overall health. Ensure you're getting an adequate amount based on your body's needs, which may change as you age.

- **Vitamins and Minerals:** These micronutrients are crucial for overall health. Look for foods rich in vitamins and minerals like calcium, vitamin D, iron, and potassium.

- **Ingredients List:** The ingredients are listed in order of quantity, from highest to lowest. Look for whole, unprocessed ingredients, and be cautious of foods with long lists of additives or artificial ingredients.

By becoming proficient in reading nutrition labels, you empower yourself to make informed decisions about what you eat, ensuring that your diet supports your health and well-being as you age. It's a testament to your care and respect for your body and its journey through the golden years.

Understanding Net Carbs and Their Importance in the Aging Body

As we embrace the golden years, the concept of net carbs becomes a vital tool in our nutritional toolkit, helping us navigate the dietary choices that best support our health and vitality. Understanding net carbs is about more than just numbers; it's about making informed decisions that respect the unique needs of our aging bodies. Let's explore the significance of net carbs and their role in maintaining well-being as we age.

The Essence of Net Carbs in Senior Nutrition

Net carbs accurately represent how carbohydrates impact our body, particularly regarding blood sugar levels and ketosis. They are calculated by subtracting fiber and certain sugar alcohols from the total carbohydrate count. This distinction is crucial for seniors, especially those following a ketogenic diet or managing diabetes, as it allows for better blood sugar control and adherence to a low-carb lifestyle.

By focusing on net carbs, seniors can enjoy a variety of nutrient-dense foods without compromising their health goals. This approach supports sustained energy levels, cognitive function, and healthy weight management—critical factors in aging gracefully and maintaining independence.

The Role of Fiber in Calculating Net Carbs

Fiber is a cornerstone of healthy aging, offering benefits like improved digestion, reduced risk of chronic diseases, and enhanced satiety. In the context of net carbs, fiber is subtracted from total carbohydrates because it has minimal impact on blood sugar levels. This adjustment allows seniors to incorporate fiber-rich foods like vegetables, nuts, and seeds into their diet without exceeding their carb limit.

Prioritizing fiber intake not only aids in managing net carbs but also supports overall digestive health and well-being. It's a gentle yet powerful way to nurture the body and promote longevity.

Navigating Sugar Alcohols in Net Carb Calculation

Sugar alcohols are commonly used as low-calorie sweeteners in sugar-free and low-carb products. While they have a lower impact on blood sugar than regular sugar, their effect can vary. For seniors, especially those with sensitive digestive systems or diabetes, it's essential to consider how sugar alcohols influence net carb calculations and overall well-being.

When calculating net carbs, some sugar alcohols can be partially subtracted, depending on their glycemic index. Being mindful of their presence in foods and their potential effects on your body allows you to enjoy sweetness in moderation without derailing your health goals.

Understanding and managing net carbs is akin to having a roadmap for nutritional well-being in the aging journey. It empowers seniors to make choices that fuel their bodies, support their minds, and bring joy to their palates, all while honoring the wisdom of their years.

CHAPTER 3:
GETTING STARTED WITH KETO

Embarking on the ketogenic journey in your golden years is like opening a new chapter in the book of life, filled with the promise of vitality and well-being. I'm here to guide you through the initial steps, ensuring your transition into this nourishing lifestyle is enjoyable and seamless. Let's delve into the essentials of setting up your keto kitchen, crafting a comprehensive shopping list, confidently dining out, and organizing your meals for success.

Setting Up Your Keto Kitchen: Essentials for Beginners

Creating a keto-friendly kitchen is akin to setting the stage for a harmonious symphony. Begin by stocking your pantry with staples like coconut oil, almond flour, and low-carb sweeteners like erythritol or stevia. Invest in quality cookware, including a non-stick skillet for perfect omelets and a slow cooker for tender meats.. Let's explore the must-haves for your keto kitchen.

1. **Essential Fats:** The cornerstone of the keto diet is healthy fats. Stock your pantry with various oils such as extra virgin olive oil, coconut oil, and avocado oil. These will be your go-to fats for cooking and adding richness to your meals. Additionally, include other sources of healthy

fats like ghee, grass-fed butter, and MCT oil for bulletproof coffee or smoothies.

2. **Quality Proteins:** Prioritize high-quality, minimally processed proteins. Look for grass-fed beef, pasture-raised poultry, wild-caught fish, and free-range eggs. These protein sources are more nutritious and align with the keto diet's emphasis on whole, unprocessed foods.

3. **Low-Carb Vegetables:** Vegetables are essential for their fiber content and micronutrients. Focus on non-starchy vegetables such as leafy greens (spinach, kale), cruciferous vegetables (broccoli, cauliflower), and other low-carb options like zucchini, bell peppers, and asparagus. These can be used in various dishes, from salads to stir-fries, adding color and nutrition to your meals.

4. **Keto-Friendly Dairy:** Opt for full-fat options for those who include dairy in their diet. Full-fat cheese, heavy cream, and sour cream can add a delicious creaminess to your dishes. If you're sensitive to dairy, look for lactose-free or dairy-free alternatives still high in fat.

5. **Pantry Staples:** Equip your pantry with keto-friendly flours like almond and coconut flour for low-carb baking. Sweeteners such as erythritol, monk fruit, and stevia can be used in moderation to satisfy sweet cravings without impacting your carb count.

6. **Snacks and Convenience Foods:** For quick snacks, stock up on olives, nuts, seeds, and cheese. Look for low-carb snack bars and shakes for on-the-go options. Be mindful of the ingredients list to ensure they fit within your keto guidelines.

7. **Herbs and Spices:** A well-stocked spice cabinet can elevate keto dishes. Fresh herbs like basil, cilantro, and rosemary add flavor without adding carbs. Spices such as cinnamon, cumin, and paprika can enhance the taste of your meals while keeping them keto-friendly.

8. **Kitchen Tools:** The right tools can make keto meal prep easier. A good quality food processor, blender, and spiralizer can help you create various keto dishes. Measuring cups and spoons, a kitchen scale, and airtight containers for storage are also essential for portion control and meal planning.

Setting up your keto kitchen with these essentials creates an environment that supports your dietary goals. Remember, the keto journey is not just about what you can't eat but about discovering the abundance of delicious, nutritious foods that fuel your body and nourish your soul. Welcome to a world of vibrant flavors and wholesome eating as you embark on this exciting path toward health and vitality.

Shopping List for Keto Beginners Over 60

As you embark on your keto journey, having a well-organized shopping list can make all the difference. Here's a comprehensive list of products to look for during your next grocery trip:

Fats and Oils	❖ Coconut Oil ❖ Olive Oil ❖ MCT Oil ❖ Grass-Fed Butter ❖ Avocado Oil
Proteins	❖ Grass-Fed Beef ❖ Free-Range Chicken ❖ Wild-Caught Salmon ❖ Eggs ❖ Pork ❖ Lamb

Dairy	❖ Full-Fat Greek Yogurt ❖ Heavy Cream ❖ Cheese (Cheddar, Mozzarella, Feta, Brie) ❖ Butter or Ghee
Low-Carb Vegetables	❖ Leafy Greens (Spinach, Kale, Arugula) ❖ Broccoli ❖ Cauliflower ❖ Zucchini ❖ Bell Peppers ❖ Asparagus ❖ Cucumbers ❖ Avocados
Nuts and Seeds	❖ Almonds ❖ Walnuts ❖ Chia Seeds ❖ Flaxseeds ❖ Pumpkin Seeds
Pantry Staples	❖ Almond Flour ❖ Coconut Flour ❖ Low-carb sweeteners (Erythritol ❖ Stevia, Monk Fruit) ❖ Canned Coconut Milk ❖ Canned Tomatoes ❖ Bone Broth
Snacks	❖ Olives ❖ Cheese Slices ❖ Pork Rinds ❖ Dark Chocolate (at least 85% cocoa)

Condiments and Spices	❖ Olive Oil-Based Salad Dressings ❖ Apple Cider Vinegar ❖ Mustard ❖ Herbs and Spices (Basil, Oregano, Cinnamon, Turmeric)
Beverages	❖ Unsweetened Almond Milk ❖ Unsweetened Coconut Milk ❖ Herbal Teas ❖ Coffee

With these items on your shopping list, you'll be well-prepared to create delicious and nutritious keto-friendly meals that cater to your dietary needs and preferences.

Tips for Dining Out on Keto: Navigating Menus as a Senior

Dining out while following a keto diet can be a delightful experience with some foresight. Look for dishes that feature grilled or roasted proteins paired with vegetables. Be cautious of hidden carbs in sauces and dressings; opting for olive oil and vinegar or asking for sauces on the side can help you stay on track. If a meal has a high-carb side like potatoes or rice, don't hesitate to request a substitution, such as extra vegetables or a side salad. Embrace the social and culinary joys of dining out, knowing that with a few simple strategies, you can enjoy a delicious meal that aligns with your keto lifestyle.

Meal Prep and Planning: Organizing Your Keto Meals

Effective meal prep and planning are the cornerstones of a successful keto diet. Start by planning your weekly meals, incorporating various protein sources, healthy fats, and low-carb vegetables to ensure balanced nutrition. Set aside time for batch cooking, preparing staples like hard-boiled eggs, grilled chicken, and roasted vegetables in advance. Use portion-control containers to store meals, making it easy to grab a keto-friendly option when you're short on time. Embrace the creativity of mixing and matching ingredients to keep your meals exciting and varied. With thoughtful meal prep and planning, you can enjoy delicious, hassle-free keto meals that support your health goals.

As you begin your keto journey, remember that each step is an opportunity to nurture your body and celebrate the richness of life. With a well-prepared kitchen, a thoughtful shopping list, the confidence to dine out, and an organized meal plan, you're setting the stage for a vibrant and healthy chapter in your life.

CHAPTERS 4:
COMMON MISTAKES AND SOLUTIONS IN KETO DIET FOR PEOPLE OVER 60

As we gracefully embrace our golden years, adopting a ketogenic lifestyle can open doors to enhanced well-being and vitality. However, the journey has its challenges. Awareness of common pitfalls and their solutions can pave the way for a smoother, more rewarding keto experience. Let's explore some frequent missteps and how to navigate them, ensuring that your path to health is as fulfilling as delicious.

Overlooking Micronutrients: The Importance of Vitamins and Minerals

While macros get the spotlight in keto, micronutrients play a crucial supporting role. A deficiency in vitamins and minerals can lead to fatigue, weakened bones, and a compromised immune system. To avoid this, diversify your diet with nutrient-rich foods like leafy greens for magnesium and iron, berries for antioxidants, and fatty fish for omega-3s and vitamin D. Consider supplementing with a high-quality multivitamin, especially if your diet lacks variety.

Neglecting Hydration: Staying Properly Hydrated

Hydration is critical to maintaining energy levels and aiding digestion, yet it's often overlooked. On keto, your body may excrete more water, making it crucial to drink enough fluids. Aim for at least 8 cups of water daily, and replenish electrolytes with foods like avocados and bone broth or a balanced electrolyte supplement. Remember, hydration is not just about water; it's about maintaining the body's balance.

Misunderstanding Fats: Choosing the Right Types of Fats

Fats are the cornerstone of the keto diet, but not all fats are beneficial. Saturated and trans fats from processed foods can harm heart health, while monounsaturated and polyunsaturated fats from sources like olive oil, nuts, and fish support it. Strike a balance by incorporating a variety of healthy fats and being mindful of portion sizes to ensure you're fueling your body with the right kind of energy.

Overcomplicating Meals: Keeping It Simple and Sustainable

The beauty of keto lies in its simplicity. Overcomplicating meals with intricate recipes or rare ingredients can lead to frustration and burnout. Embrace the elegance of simplicity by focusing on whole, unprocessed foods. Create meals around a protein source, add various low-carb vegetables, and incorporate healthy fats for flavor and satiety. This approach not only makes meal prep more manageable but also more enjoyable.

Underestimating the Importance of Sleep: Rest and Recovery

Quality sleep is vital for overall health, especially for those on a keto diet. Lack of sleep can disrupt ketosis, increase cravings, and lead to weight gain. Prioritize sleep by establishing a regular bedtime routine, creating a comfortable sleep environment, and avoiding caffeine and screens before bed. Remember, restful sleep is a crucial ingredient for a healthy, balanced life.

By being mindful of these common mistakes and implementing their solutions, you can enhance your keto journey, making it a delightful and nourishing experience. Embrace each day with the knowledge that you are taking steps to support your health and well-being in the most golden years of your life.

CHAPTERS 5:
CONTROLLING MEDICAL PARAMETERS ON KETO

As we navigate the waters of the ketogenic lifestyle, particularly in our later years, it becomes imperative to monitor and manage critical medical parameters. This vigilant approach ensures that our keto journey is effective for weight management and energy levels and conducive to our overall health and well-being.

Monitoring Blood Sugar Levels: Key for Diabetics

Understanding the Impact of Keto on Blood Sugar

The ketogenic diet's low carbohydrate content can significantly change blood sugar levels. Reducing the body's carbohydrate intake diminishes the need for insulin, promoting more stable blood sugar levels. This stability is particularly beneficial for individuals with diabetes or prediabetes, as it can help in managing the condition more effectively.

Tips for Measuring and Managing Blood Sugar

Regular blood sugar level monitoring is crucial for individuals on a keto diet, especially for those with diabetes. Utilize a reliable glucose meter to check your levels consistently, noting how different foods and activities affect your readings. Collaborate with your healthcare provider to tailor your diet and medication to your needs, ensuring a safe and effective approach to managing your blood sugar.

Managing Blood Pressure: Heart Health on Keto

The Effect of Keto on Blood Pressure

The ketogenic diet may positively affect blood pressure due to its potential impact on weight loss, insulin sensitivity, and inflammation reduction. Weight loss can alleviate pressure on blood vessels, while improved insulin sensitivity can aid in vascular relaxation, contributing to healthier blood pressure levels.

Strategies for Maintaining Healthy Blood Pressure

To support healthy blood pressure on a keto diet:

1. Incorporate a diverse range of nutrient-dense foods, including leafy greens, avocados, and fatty fish, which are rich in potassium and omega-3 fatty acids.

2. Maintain adequate hydration and limit sodium intake by choosing fresh, whole foods over processed alternatives.

3. Complement your dietary efforts with regular physical activity and stress-reducing practices to promote optimal blood pressure further.

Lipid Profile and Cholesterol: Navigating Changes

Interpreting Changes in Cholesterol Levels

Adopting a ketogenic diet can alter your lipid profile, including levels of total cholesterol, HDL (good cholesterol), LDL (bad cholesterol), and triglycerides. While some individuals may experience an increase in LDL cholesterol, others may observe improvements in HDL and triglyceride levels, which benefit heart health.

Adjusting Your Keto Diet for Optimal Lipid Health

If concerns arise regarding your cholesterol levels on a keto diet, focus on incorporating heart-healthy fats such as those found in olive oil, nuts, and seeds. Opt for lean protein sources and increase your consumption of fibrous vegetables to support overall lipid health. Regular consultations with your healthcare provider are essential to monitor your lipid profile and make any necessary dietary adjustments.

When embarking on the keto journey, especially as we age, it's essential to maintain a delicate balance that aligns with our lifestyle goals and safeguards our health. By monitoring and managing these critical medical parameters, we ensure that our path to wellness is informed and holistic, paving the way for a journey filled with vitality and longevity.

CHAPTERS 6:
OVERCOMING CHALLENGES FOR BEGINNERS

Embarking on the keto journey, especially in the later stages of life, can be akin to navigating a new landscape filled with excitement and challenges. As a nutritional specialist, I understand the hurdles that may arise and am here to provide guidance and support to help you gracefully overcome them. Let's explore some common challenges beginners face and discover strategies to navigate these easily and confidently.

Breaking Through Weight Loss Plateaus: Tips for Older Dieters

Reaching a weight loss plateau can be disheartening, but it's a natural part of the journey. To break through, consider mixing up your routine by varying your physical activity or adjusting your calorie intake. Intermittent fasting, when done safely, can also be an effective tool to reignite weight loss. Patience and persistence are key; small, consistent changes can lead to significant long-term results.

Handling Cravings and Social Situations: Advice for Beginners

Cravings and social gatherings can present challenges for those new to the keto lifestyle. To manage cravings:

1. Ensure you're eating nutrient-dense meals that keep you satiated and have keto-friendly snacks on hand.

2. When attending social events, plan by eating a satisfying meal beforehand or bringing a keto-friendly dish to share.

3. Embrace these situations as opportunities to explore new foods and share your journey with others.

Staying Motivated: Setting Realistic Goals and Celebrating Success

Staying motivated is crucial for long-term success on the keto diet. Set realistic, achievable goals that align with your lifestyle and health objectives. Celebrate your accomplishments, no matter how small, to maintain a positive mindset. Surround yourself with a supportive community, whether online or in person, to share experiences and encourage each other.

Dealing with Keto Flu: Symptoms and Remedies

The keto flu is a common challenge for beginners, characterized by symptoms like fatigue, headaches, and irritability. These temporary symptoms can be mitigated by staying hydrated, replenishing electrolytes, and ensuring adequate rest. Gradually easing into the keto diet can also help your body adjust comfortably.

Overcoming the challenges of the keto diet is a journey of self-discovery and resilience. Embrace each obstacle as an opportunity to learn and grow, knowing that you're moving closer to a healthier, more vibrant you with each step. Remember, the path to wellness is a marathon, not a sprint, and every challenge overcome is a testament to your dedication and strength.

CHAPTERS 7:
EXERCISE AND KETO FOR BEGINNERS

Embarking on a ketogenic lifestyle is a beautiful journey toward health and vitality, especially as we age. However, regular exercise is vital to genuinely embracing this lifestyle's benefits. As we explore the world of fitness alongside keto, let's focus on gentle, practical exercises that complement our dietary choices and enhance our overall well-being.

Safe Exercises for Older Adults: Low-Impact Options

As we age, finding low-impact exercises that are gentle on the joints yet effective in maintaining fitness becomes essential. Consider incorporating:

- **Walking:** A simple yet powerful way to stay active.

- **Swimming:** Provides a full-body workout with minimal joint strain.

- **Tai Chi:** Improves balance, flexibility, and mental well-being.

- **Yoga:** Enhances flexibility, strength, and relaxation.

- **Cycling:** A great cardio workout with a low impact on the knees.

These activities offer a balanced approach to fitness, ensuring that you stay active without overexerting yourself.

Combining Keto with Exercise: Strategies for Beginners

Merging a keto diet with an exercise routine can be highly rewarding. To maximize the benefits:

- **Stay Hydrated:** Keep your fluid intake up to support exercise performance.

- **Monitor Your Energy Levels:** Adjust your activity intensity based on your feelings.

- **Time Your Meals:** Consider eating a small, balanced meal a few hours before exercising.

- **Listen to Your Body:** Start slow and gradually increase intensity as you become more comfortable.

By synchronizing your diet and exercise, you can achieve a harmonious balance that supports your health goals.

Daily Routines for Active Living: Staying Fit and Flexible

Incorporating movement into your daily routine is a simple yet effective way to maintain fitness:

- **Morning Stretches:** Start your day with gentle stretching to awaken your body.

- **Take Frequent Breaks:** If you sit for long periods, stand up and move around regularly.

- **Use the Stairs:** Opt for stairs over elevators when possible.

- **Evening Walks:** End your day with a leisurely walk to unwind and stay active.

Integrating these small movements into your day allows you to keep your body active and flexible.

Tailoring Your Exercise Routine to Your Fitness Level

Creating an exercise routine that aligns with your fitness level is crucial for both safety and enjoyment:

- **Assess Your Current Fitness:** Be honest about your starting point and set realistic goals.

- **Choose Appropriate Activities:** Select exercises that match your abilities and interests.

- **Progress Gradually:** Increase the intensity and duration of your workouts slowly over time.

- **Seek Professional Guidance:** Consult a fitness trainer or physical therapist for personalized advice.

You can enjoy a fulfilling and sustainable fitness journey by tailoring your routine to your needs.

4-Week Exercise Plan: Getting Started with Fitness

Embarking on a new exercise regimen can be daunting, but a structured plan can help ease the transition:

- **Week 1:** Focus on gentle activities like walking or swimming for 15-20 minutes daily.
- **Week 2:** Introduce light strength training with resistance bands or bodyweight exercises.
- **Week 3:** Increase your cardio duration to 30 minutes and add more variety to your strength training.
- **Week 4:** Explore new activities like yoga or cycling and improve your progress.

By following this gradual approach, you can build a solid foundation for fitness that complements your keto lifestyle.

Incorporating exercise into your keto journey is like adding music to a dance—it enhances the experience and brings a new level of joy and vitality. With these gentle, practical strategies, you can create a balanced routine supporting your health and well-being for years.

Here's a detailed 4-week Exercise Plan designed for beginners, especially those over 60, to help you get started with fitness alongside your keto journey:

WEEK 1: INTRODUCTION TO MOVEMENT	
Day 1	15-minute walk at a comfortable pace.
Day 2	Rest or gentle stretching for 10 minutes.
Day 3	15-minute walk, a slightly faster pace than Day 1.
Day 4	Rest or 10 minutes of gentle yoga focusing on breath and balance.

Day 5	20-minute walk at a comfortable pace.
Day 6	Rest or 10 minutes of light stretching.
Day 7	15-minute leisurely walk.

WEEK 2: BUILDING CONSISTENCY

Day 1	20-minute walk, incorporating some inclines if possible.
Day 2	Rest or 10 minutes of gentle yoga focusing on flexibility.
Day 3	20-minute walk, maintain a steady pace.
Day 4	Rest or 10 minutes of stretching, focusing on the legs and lower back.
Day 5	25-minute walk; try to include different terrains.
Day 6	Rest or 10 minutes of balance exercises (e.g., standing on one foot, tai chi moves).
Day 7	20-minute leisurely walk.

WEEK 3: INTRODUCING VARIETY

Day 1	30-minute walk; aim for a brisk pace.
Day 2	Rest or 15 minutes of yoga, including strength poses.
Day 3	15-minute swim or water aerobics session.

Day 4	Rest or 15 minutes of stretching focusing on upper body.
Day 5	30-minute walk with intervals (2 minutes fast, 3 minutes slow).
Day 6	Rest or 15 minutes of gentle tai chi.
Day 7	25-minute leisurely walk in nature.

WEEK 4: INCREASING INTENSITY

Day 1	35-minute walk with intervals (3 minutes fast, 2 minutes slow).
Day 2	Rest or 20 minutes of yoga, incorporating more challenging poses.
Day 3	20-minute swim or water aerobics with some light resistance.
Day 4	Rest or 20 minutes of stretching, focusing on full-body flexibility.
Day 5	40-minute walk, maintaining a brisk pace throughout.
Day 6	Rest or 20 minutes of balance and strength exercises (e.g., leg lifts, wall push-ups).
Day 7	30-minute leisurely walk to unwind and reflect on your progress.

Throughout this 4-week plan, listen to your body and adjust the intensity and duration of the exercises as needed. Stay hydrated, especially after exercising, and ensure you're fueling your body with nutritious keto-friendly meals to support your fitness journey. Remember, the goal is to gradually build your strength and endurance while enjoying the process.

To effectively repeat this 4-week exercise plan for three months, here are some recommendations to keep in mind:

Month 1: Foundation Building

- **Focus:** Use the first month to establish a solid foundation. Stick closely to the outlined plan, paying attention to your body's responses.

- **Adjustments:** If any exercises feel too easy or too challenging, make minor adjustments to the intensity or duration.

- **Reflection:** At the end of the month, reflect on what worked well and any areas where you faced challenges.

Month 2: Progress and Variety

- **Progress:** Aim to increase the intensity or duration of your exercises gradually. For example, add 5 minutes to your walks or include more challenging resistance exercises.

- **Variety:** Introduce new activities to keep your routine interesting. Consider adding a new exercise class, such as water aerobics or Pilates, once a week.

- **Mind-Body Connection:** Incorporate more mind-body exercises, such as yoga or tai chi, to enhance balance, flexibility, and mental well-being.

Month 3: Consistency and Challenges

- **Consistency:** Focus on maintaining a consistent exercise routine for steady progress.

- **Challenges:** Introduce small challenges to keep yourself motivated. This could be a slightly longer walk, a new yoga pose, or an extra set of resistance exercises.

- **Celebration:** Celebrate your achievements and the progress you've made over the three months. Recognize the positive changes in your fitness and overall well-being.

General Tips:

1. **Listen to Your Body:** Always listen to your body and modify the exercises if needed. Rest when necessary, and avoid pushing yourself too hard.

2. **Stay Hydrated:** Keep yourself well-hydrated, especially on exercise days.

3. **Nutrition:** Ensure your diet supports your exercise routine, focusing on nutritious, keto-friendly foods.

4. **Support:** Consider finding a workout buddy or joining a group class for additional motivation and support.

5. **Regular Check-ins:** Schedule regular check-ins with yourself or a fitness professional to assess your progress and make necessary adjustments to your routine.

By following these recommendations and adapting the plan to your evolving fitness levels and preferences, you can effectively repeat this 4-week exercise plan for three months, leading to sustained improvements in your health and fitness.

CHAPTERS 8:
FAQS FOR KETO BEGINNERS

Embarking on the ketogenic journey is an adventure filled with discoveries and learning. As a nutritional specialist, I understand that beginners, especially older adults, may have questions and concerns. This section addresses common queries, debunking myths, and providing guidance to ensure a smooth and enjoyable keto experience.

Answers to Common Questions from Older Adults

Q: Is the keto diet safe for older adults?

A: When done correctly, the keto diet can be safe and beneficial for older adults. Focusing on nutrient-dense foods and consulting a healthcare provider to ensure the diet is tailored to your specific health needs is essential.

Q: Can keto help with weight loss in older adults?

A: Absolutely. The keto diet can be an effective way to lose weight by promoting fat-burning and reducing appetite. However, weight loss should be approached gradually, and overall nutrition should remain a priority.

Q: How can I get enough nutrients on a keto diet?

A: Focus on incorporating a variety of low-carb vegetables, high-quality proteins, and healthy fats into your meals. Consider supplementing with vitamins and minerals if needed, and stay hydrated.

Q: Can the keto diet improve energy levels in older adults?

A: Many people find that the keto diet enhances their energy levels by providing a steady fuel source in ketones. To support your energy levels, ensure you eat balanced meals and get adequate rest.

Debunking Keto Myths: What Beginners Need to Know

Myth 1: Keto is just a high-protein diet.

Fact: The keto diet is high in fat, moderate in protein, and low in carbohydrates. Protein intake should be adequate but not excessive.

Myth 2: Keto means cutting out all carbs.

Fact: While the keto diet does restrict carbs, it allows for a moderate intake of low-carb vegetables and some fruits, providing essential nutrients and fiber.

Myth 3: The keto diet is bad for your heart.

Fact: When done correctly, focusing on healthy fats and avoiding processed foods, the keto diet can support heart health.

Myth 4: You can't eat any fruits or vegetables on keto.

Fact: The keto diet encourages the consumption of many low-carb vegetables and some fruits, like berries, for their nutritional value.

Navigating Challenges and Concerns

Challenge: Dealing with the keto flu.

Solution: Stay hydrated, replenish electrolytes, and ease into the diet gradually to minimize symptoms.

Challenge: Managing social situations.

Solution: Plan by eating before events, bringing keto-friendly dishes, or choosing restaurants with suitable options.

Challenge: Staying consistent.

Solution: Set realistic goals, track progress, and celebrate small victories to stay motivated.

Challenge: Overcoming cravings.

Solution: Keep keto-friendly snacks on hand, find low-carb alternatives to your favorite treats, and ensure you eat satisfying meals.

I aim to provide clarity and confidence to those embarking on the keto journey by addressing these FAQs. Remember, every individual's experience is unique, and it's essential to listen to your body and make adjustments as needed to ensure a healthy and enjoyable journey.

CHAPTERS 9: RECIPES

BREAKFAST

Spinach and Feta Omelet

🍽 **Yield:** 2 servings

🕐 **Prep time:** 5 minutes

🎩 **Cook time:** 7 minutes

NUTRITIONAL INFORMATION (PER SERVING)

* Calories: 300
* Fat: 23g
* Protein: 18g
* Net Carbs: 2g
* Fiber: 1g

TIPS

* *You can customize your omelet with other keto-friendly ingredients, such as mushrooms, bell peppers, or cooked bacon.*

* *Add a splash of heavy cream to the eggs before whisking for a fluffier omelet.*

* *Pair your omelet with a side of avocado slices for an extra dose of healthy fats.*

INGREDIENTS

- ☐ *2 large eggs*
- ☐ *1 cup fresh spinach, chopped*
- ☐ *1/4 cup feta cheese, crumbled*
- ☐ *1 tablespoon olive oil*
- ☐ *Salt and pepper to taste*

INSTRUCTIONS

1. Whisk the eggs with salt and pepper in a mixing bowl until well combined.

2. Heat olive oil in a non-stick skillet over medium heat.

3. Add the chopped spinach to the skillet and sauté for 1-2 minutes until slightly wilted.

4. Pour the whisked eggs over the spinach, covering it evenly.

5. Sprinkle crumbled feta cheese on top of the eggs.

6. Cover the skillet with a lid and cook for 3-4 minutes until the eggs are set and the cheese slightly melts.

7. Gently fold the omelet in half and slide it onto a plate.

8. Serve warm and enjoy!

Keto Avocado Toast

🍽 **Yield:** 2 servings

🕐 **Prep time:** 5 minutes

🍞 **Cook time:** 2 minutes

NUTRITIONAL INFORMATION (PER SERVING)

- ❖ Calories: 320
- ❖ Fat: 28g
- ❖ Protein: 6g
- ❖ Net Carbs: 4g
- ❖ Fiber: 8g

TIPS

- ❖ *Add a sprinkle of red pepper flakes or a squeeze of lemon juice on top of the avocado toast for extra flavor.*

- ❖ *Top the avocado toast with a poached or fried egg if you want more protein.*

INGREDIENTS

- ☐ *1 large avocado*
- ☐ *2 slices keto-friendly bread*
- ☐ *1 tablespoon olive oil*
- ☐ *Salt and pepper to taste*

INSTRUCTIONS

1. Toast the keto-friendly bread slices until golden brown.

2. Mash the avocado in a bowl and season with salt and pepper.

3. Spread the mashed avocado evenly on the toasted bread slices.

4. Drizzle olive oil over the avocado.

5. Serve immediately and enjoy!

Keto Berry Smoothie

🍽 **Yield:** 2 servings

🕐 **Prep time:** 5 minutes

🍞 **Cook time:** 0 minutes

NUTRITIONAL INFORMATION (PER SERVING)

- ❖ Calories: 150
- ❖ Fat: 7g
- ❖ Protein: 6g
- ❖ Net Carbs: 8g
- ❖ Fiber: 4g

TIPS

- ❖ *For added creaminess, include a tablespoon of almond butter or coconut cream in the smoothie.*

- ❖ *If you prefer a sweeter smoothie, adjust the amount of erythritol to your taste or add a few drops of liquid stevia.*

INGREDIENTS

- ☐ *1/2 cup unsweetened almond milk*
- ☐ *1/2 cup mixed berries (strawberries, raspberries, blueberries)*
- ☐ *1/4 cup Greek yogurt (full-fat)*
- ☐ *1 tablespoon chia seeds*
- ☐ *1 tablespoon erythritol (optional)*
- ☐ *Ice cubes*

INSTRUCTIONS

1. Combine almond milk, berries, Greek yogurt, chia seeds, and erythritol (if using) in a blender.

2. Blend until smooth, adding ice cubes for desired thickness.

3. Pour the smoothie into a glass and serve cold.

Keto Egg Muffins

🍽️ **Yield:** 6 servings

🕐 **Prep time:** 10 minutes

🧁 **Cook time:** 20 minutes

NUTRITIONAL INFORMATION (PER MUFFIN)

- ❖ Calories: 120
- ❖ Fat: 9g
- ❖ Protein: 9g
- ❖ Net Carbs: 1g
- ❖ Fiber: 0g

TIPS

- ❖ *Feel free to customize the egg muffins with your favorite keto-friendly vegetables or cooked meats.*

- ❖ *These egg muffins can be stored in the refrigerator for up to 4 days or frozen for extended storage. Reheat in the microwave for a quick and easy breakfast.*

INGREDIENTS

- ☐ *6 large eggs*
- ☐ *1/2 cup cooked bacon, chopped*
- ☐ *1/2 cup shredded cheddar cheese*
- ☐ *1/4 cup diced bell peppers*
- ☐ *Salt and pepper to taste*

INSTRUCTIONS

1. Preheat the oven to 375°F and grease a muffin tin.

2. In a bowl, whisk the eggs and season with salt and pepper.

3. Divide the bacon, cheese, and bell peppers evenly among the muffin cups.

4. Pour the whisked eggs over the filling in each cup.

5. Bake for 15-20 minutes or until the egg muffins are set and lightly golden.

6. Let cool for a few minutes before removing from the tin and serving.

Keto Chia Seed Pudding

🍽 **Yield:** 2 servings

🕐 **Prep time:** 5 minutes

🍞 **Cook time:** 0 minutes (plus at least 2 hours chilling)

NUTRITIONAL INFORMATION (PER SERVING)

* Calories: 180
* Fat: 12g
* Protein: 5g
* Net Carbs: 2g
* Fiber: 10g

TIPS

* *Blend the mixture before refrigerating to break down the chia seeds for a smoother texture.*

* *Get creative with your toppings! For extra flavor, try adding a dollop of almond butter, a sprinkle of cinnamon, or a few cacao nibs.*

INGREDIENTS

- ☐ *1/4 cup chia seeds*
- ☐ *1 cup unsweetened almond milk*
- ☐ *1/2 teaspoon vanilla extract*
- ☐ *1 tablespoon erythritol or sweetener of choice*
- ☐ *Optional toppings: nuts, berries, or unsweetened coconut flakes*

INSTRUCTIONS

1. Mix chia seeds, almond milk, vanilla extract, and erythritol in a bowl.

2. Stir well and let sit for 5 minutes, then stir again to prevent clumping.

3. Cover and refrigerate for at least 2 hours or overnight until thickened.

4. Serve with your choice of toppings.

Keto Sausage and Spinach Breakfast Skillet

🍽 **Yield:** 4 servings

🕐 **Prep time:** 5 minutes

🍞 **Cook time:** 15 minutes

NUTRITIONAL INFORMATION (PER SERVING)

- ❖ Calories: 250
- ❖ Fat: 19g
- ❖ Protein: 17g
- ❖ Net Carbs: 1g
- ❖ Fiber: 0.5g

TIPS

- ❖ *Add diced bell peppers or mushrooms to the skillet with the sausage and spinach to make this dish even heartier.*

- ❖ *If you're not a fan of runny yolks, cook the eggs until they reach your desired level of doneness.*

INGREDIENTS

- ☐ *4 breakfast sausage links (sugar-free)*
- ☐ *2 cups fresh spinach*
- ☐ *4 large eggs*
- ☐ *1 tablespoon olive oil*
- ☐ *Salt and pepper to taste*
- ☐ *Optional: shredded cheese for topping*

INSTRUCTIONS

1. Heat olive oil in a skillet over medium heat.
2. Add sausage links and cook until browned and fully cooked.
3. Add spinach to the skillet and sauté until wilted.
4. Make four wells in the mixture and crack an egg into each.
5. Cover the skillet and cook until the egg whites are set but the yolks are still runny.
6. Season with salt and pepper and sprinkle with cheese if desired.
7. Serve hot directly from the skillet.

LUNCH

Keto Chicken Caesar Salad

🍴 **Yield:** 2 servings

🕐 **Prep time:** 15 minutes

🍞 **Cook time:** 10 minutes

NUTRITIONAL INFORMATION (PER SERVING)

- ❖ Calories: 450
- ❖ Fat: 35g
- ❖ Protein: 30g
- ❖ Net Carbs: 4g
- ❖ Fiber: 2g

TIPS

- ❖ *For added crunch, sprinkle some pumpkin seeds or chopped almonds on top of the salad.*

- ❖ *Make this salad ahead of time for a quick and easy lunch option. Store the dressing separately and toss it with the salad just before serving.*

INGREDIENTS

- [ ] *2 boneless, skinless chicken breasts*
- [ ] *4 cups chopped romaine lettuce*
- [ ] *1/4 cup grated Parmesan cheese*
- [ ] *1/2 cup Caesar dressing (keto-friendly)*
- [ ] *1 tablespoon olive oil*
- [ ] *Salt and pepper to taste*
- [ ] *Optional: 2 tablespoons keto-friendly croutons*

INSTRUCTIONS

1. Season the chicken breasts with salt and pepper.

2. Heat olive oil in a skillet over medium heat. Cook the chicken for 5 minutes on each side or until fully cooked. Let it rest for a few minutes, then slice it.

3. In a large bowl, toss the chopped romaine lettuce with Caesar dressing until evenly coated.

4. Divide the dressed lettuce between two plates. Top with sliced chicken and sprinkle with Parmesan cheese.

5. Add keto-friendly croutons if desired and serve immediately.

Keto BLT Lettuce Wrap

🍽 **Yield:** 2 servings

🕐 **Prep time:** 10 minutes

🍞 **Cook time:** 10 minutes

NUTRITIONAL INFORMATION (PER SERVING)

* Calories: 380
* Fat: 34g
* Protein: 12g
* Net Carbs: 3g
* Fiber: 1g

TIPS

* *For a more filling wrap, add some sliced grilled chicken or turkey.*
* *If you're on the go, wrap these in parchment paper for an easy, mess-free lunch option.*

INGREDIENTS

- [ ] *4 large lettuce leaves (e.g., romaine or iceberg)*
- [ ] *8 slices bacon, cooked until crispy*
- [ ] *1 medium tomato, sliced*
- [ ] *1/4 cup mayonnaise (keto-friendly)*
- [ ] *Salt and pepper to taste*
- [ ] *Optional: sliced avocado or a sprinkle of cheese*

INSTRUCTIONS

1. Lay the lettuce leaves on a flat surface.

2. Spread a tablespoon of mayonnaise on each lettuce leaf.

3. Place two slices of bacon and a few tomato slices on each lettuce leaf.

4. Season with salt and pepper, and add any additional toppings you like.

5. Roll up the lettuce leaves to enclose the fillings and secure them with a toothpick.

6. Serve immediately and enjoy your keto-friendly BLT wraps!

Keto Tuna Salad Stuffed Avocados

🍽 **Yield:** 2 servings

🕐 **Prep time:** 10 minutes

🍞 **Cook time:** 0 minutes

NUTRITIONAL INFORMATION (PER SERVING)

* Calories: 350
* Fat: 28g
* Protein: 18g
* Net Carbs: 4g
* Fiber: 7g

TIPS

* *Mix some chopped cucumber or bell pepper into the tuna salad for added crunch.*

* *Save the scooped-out avocado flesh and use it as a smoothie or a spread for another meal.*

INGREDIENTS

- ☐ *1 can (5 oz) tuna in water, drained*
- ☐ *2 avocados, halved and pitted*
- ☐ *2 tablespoons mayonnaise (keto-friendly)*
- ☐ *1 tablespoon diced celery*
- ☐ *1 tablespoon diced red onion*
- ☐ *Salt and pepper to taste*
- ☐ *Optional: a squeeze of lemon juice or a sprinkle of paprika*

INSTRUCTIONS

1. Mix the tuna, mayonnaise, celery, and red onion in a bowl. Season with salt and pepper (and lemon juice if using).

2. Scoop out some of the flesh from each avocado half to create a space for the tuna salad.

3. Fill each avocado half with the tuna salad mixture.

4. Sprinkle with paprika for added color and flavor if desired.

5. Serve immediately and enjoy your creamy, satisfying keto lunch!

Keto Shrimp and Avocado Salad

🍽 **Yield:** 2 servings

🕐 **Prep time:** 15 minutes

🎩 **Cook time:** 5 minutes

NUTRITIONAL INFORMATION (PER SERVING)

- ❖ Calories: 350
- ❖ Fat: 25g
- ❖ Protein: 25g
- ❖ Net Carbs: 6g
- ❖ Fiber: 7g

TIPS

- ❖ *For added flavor, marinate the shrimp in a mixture of lime juice, garlic, and spices before cooking.*

- ❖ *If you prefer a creamier salad, mix some of the avocado into the dressing.*

- ❖ *This salad can be customized with your favorite keto-friendly vegetables or toppings.*

INGREDIENTS

- ☐ *1/2 lb shrimp, peeled and deveined*
- ☐ *1 large avocado, diced*
- ☐ *2 cups mixed salad greens*
- ☐ *1/2 cup cherry tomatoes, halved*
- ☐ *1/4 cup cucumber, sliced*
- ☐ *2 tablespoons olive oil*
- ☐ *1 tablespoon lime juice*
- ☐ *Salt and pepper to taste*
- ☐ *Optional: cilantro, red pepper flakes*

INSTRUCTIONS

1. Heat 1 tablespoon olive oil in a skillet over medium heat. Add shrimp, season with salt and pepper, and cook until pink and opaque.

2. Combine the salad greens, cherry tomatoes, cucumber, and diced avocado in a large bowl.

3. Whisk together the remaining olive oil, lime juice, and optional seasonings in a small bowl.

4. Toss the salad with the dressing, then top with cooked shrimp.

5. Serve immediately and enjoy!

Keto Beef and Broccoli Stir-Fry

🍽 **Yield:** 2 servings

🕐 **Prep time:** 10 minutes

🍞 **Cook time:** 10 minutes

NUTRITIONAL INFORMATION (PER SERVING)

- ❖ Calories: 350
- ❖ Fat: 25g
- ❖ Protein: 25g
- ❖ Net Carbs: 5g
- ❖ Fiber: 2g

TIPS

- ❖ *Add a dash of red pepper flakes or a drizzle of chili oil for a spicier stir-fry.*

- ❖ *You can substitute the beef with chicken or shrimp for a different protein option.*

- ❖ *Serve the stir-fry over cauliflower rice for a complete keto-friendly meal.*

INGREDIENTS

- ☐ *1/2 lb beef sirloin, thinly sliced*
- ☐ *2 cups broccoli florets*
- ☐ *2 tablespoons olive oil*
- ☐ *2 cloves garlic, minced*
- ☐ *1 tablespoon soy sauce (or coconut aminos for a soy-free option)*
- ☐ *1 tablespoon sesame oil*
- ☐ *1 teaspoon ginger, grated*
- ☐ *Salt and pepper to taste*
- ☐ *Optional: sesame seeds, green onions for garnish*

INSTRUCTIONS

1. Heat 1 tablespoon olive oil in a large skillet or wok over medium-high heat.

2. Add the thinly sliced beef to the skillet and season with salt and pepper. Stir-fry until browned and cooked through, about 3-4 minutes. Remove the meat from the skillet and set aside.

3. In the same skillet, add the remaining olive oil and broccoli florets. Stir-fry for 2-3 minutes until the broccoli is tender but still crisp.

4. Add the minced garlic and grated ginger to the skillet and cook for an additional minute until fragrant.

5. Return the cooked beef to the skillet. Add soy sauce (or coconut aminos) and sesame oil. Stir everything together and cook for another 1-2 minutes.

6. Taste and adjust seasoning if necessary. Garnish with sesame seeds and sliced green onions if desired.

7. Serve immediately and enjoy!

DINNER

Keto Lemon Garlic Butter Salmon

🍽 **Yield:** 2 servings

🕐 **Prep time:** 10 minutes

🍞 **Cook time:** 15 minutes

NUTRITIONAL INFORMATION (PER SERVING)

- ❖ Calories: 350
- ❖ Fat: 24g
- ❖ Protein: 30g
- ❖ Net Carbs: 1g
- ❖ Fiber: 0g

TIPS

- ❖ *Serve the salmon with steamed asparagus or sautéed spinach for a keto-friendly meal.*

- ❖ *For added flavor, add a sprinkle of capers or a few slices of lemon on top of the salmon before baking.*

INGREDIENTS

- ☐ *2 salmon fillets (6 oz each)*
- ☐ *2 tablespoons unsalted butter*
- ☐ *2 cloves garlic, minced*
- ☐ *1 tablespoon lemon juice*
- ☐ *1 teaspoon lemon zest*
- ☐ *Salt and pepper to taste*
- ☐ *Fresh parsley, chopped for garnish*

INSTRUCTIONS

1. Preheat the oven to 375°F (190°C).

2. Season the salmon fillets with salt and pepper.

3. In a small saucepan, melt the butter over medium heat. Add the minced garlic and cook until fragrant, about 1 minute.

4. Stir in the lemon juice and lemon zest.

5. Place the salmon fillets in a baking dish and pour the lemon garlic butter over them.

6. Bake in the preheated oven for 12-15 minutes or until the salmon flakes easily with a fork.

7. Garnish with chopped parsley and serve.

Keto Creamy Garlic Chicken

🍽 **Yield:** 2 servings

🕐 **Prep time:** 10 minutes

🍞 **Cook time:** 20 minutes

NUTRITIONAL INFORMATION (PER SERVING)

- ❖ Calories: 400
- ❖ Fat: 28g
- ❖ Protein: 35g
- ❖ Net Carbs: 2g
- ❖ Fiber: 0g

TIPS

- ❖ *Pair the creamy garlic chicken with a cauliflower mash or zucchini noodles for a satisfying keto dinner.*

- ❖ *Add a pinch of red pepper flakes to the sauce for a bit of heat.*

INGREDIENTS

- [ ] *2 boneless, skinless chicken breasts*
- [ ] *1 tablespoon olive oil*
- [ ] *1/2 cup heavy cream*
- [ ] *2 cloves garlic, minced*
- [ ] *1/4 cup grated Parmesan cheese*
- [ ] *Salt and pepper to taste*
- [ ] *Fresh thyme or parsley, chopped for garnish*

INSTRUCTIONS

1. Season the chicken breasts with salt and pepper.

2. Heat the olive oil in a skillet over medium heat. Add the chicken and cook until golden brown on both sides, about 5-7 minutes per side. Remove the chicken from the skillet and set aside.

3. In the same skillet, add the minced garlic and cook until fragrant, about 1 minute.

4. Stir in the heavy cream and Parmesan cheese. Simmer for a few minutes until the sauce thickens.

5. Return the chicken to the skillet and coat it with the creamy garlic sauce.

6. Garnish with fresh thyme or parsley and serve.

Keto Beef and Mushroom Stroganoff

🍽 **Yield:** 2 servings

🕑 **Prep time:** 10 minutes

🍞 **Cook time:** 15 minutes

NUTRITIONAL INFORMATION (PER SERVING)

* Calories: 400
* Fat: 28g
* Protein: 32g
* Net Carbs: 5g
* Fiber: 1g

TIPS

* *For a more tender beef stroganoff, consider using beef tenderloin or sirloin tips instead of sirloin steak. These cuts are more tender and will cook faster.*

* *If you like a thicker sauce, you can add a small amount of cream cheese or sour cream to the stroganoff just before serving. This will give the sauce a richer, creamier texture.*

* *To boost the stroganoff's flavor, try sautéing the mushrooms in a separate pan until golden brown before adding them to the stroganoff. This will add a deeper, more complex flavor.*

INGREDIENTS

- ☐ *1/2 lb beef sirloin, thinly sliced*
- ☐ *1 cup mushrooms, sliced*
- ☐ *1/2 cup beef broth*
- ☐ *1/4 cup sour cream*
- ☐ *1 tablespoon Dijon mustard*
- ☐ *2 tablespoons olive oil*
- ☐ *1 clove garlic, minced*
- ☐ *Salt and pepper to taste*
- ☐ *Fresh parsley, chopped for garnish*

INSTRUCTIONS

1. Heat olive oil in a skillet over medium-high heat. Add the beef and cook until browned, about 3-4 minutes. Remove the meat from the skillet and set aside.

2. Add the mushrooms and garlic to the same skillet. Cook until the mushrooms are tender, about 5 minutes.

3. Stir in the beef broth and Dijon mustard. Bring to a simmer and cook for a few minutes.

4. Reduce the heat to low and stir in the sour cream—season with salt and pepper.

5. Return the beef to the skillet and stir to combine with the sauce.

6. Garnish with chopped parsley, and serve the stroganoff over cauliflower rice or zucchini noodles.

Keto Lemon Herb Roasted Chicken

🍽 **Yield:** 2 servings

🕐 **Prep time:** 10 minutes

🎩 **Cook time:** 45 minutes

NUTRITIONAL INFORMATION (PER SERVING)

- Calories: 380
- Fat: 28g
- Protein: 30g
- Net Carbs: 1g
- Fiber: 0g

TIPS

- *For added flavor depth, stuff the chicken cavity with additional lemon slices, fresh herbs, and garlic cloves before roasting.*

- *To ensure even cooking and crispy skin, pat the chicken dry with paper towels before seasoning and roasting.*

- *If you have a meat thermometer, use it to check the internal temperature of the chicken. It should reach 165°F (74°C) in the thickest part of the thigh for safe consumption.*

INGREDIENTS

- ☐ *2 chicken leg quarters (thigh and drumstick)*
- ☐ *2 tablespoons olive oil*
- ☐ *1 lemon, sliced*
- ☐ *2 cloves garlic, minced*
- ☐ *1 teaspoon dried rosemary*
- ☐ *1 teaspoon dried thyme*
- ☐ *Salt and pepper to taste*

INSTRUCTIONS

1. Preheat the oven to 400°F (200°C).

2. Rub the chicken leg quarters with olive oil, garlic, rosemary, thyme, salt, and pepper.

3. Place the chicken in a baking dish and arrange lemon slices around it.

4. Roast in the preheated oven for 45 minutes or until the chicken is cooked through and the skin is crispy.

5. Serve the roasted chicken with the lemon slices, and enjoy!

Keto Pork Chops with Creamy Mushroom Sauce

🍽 **Yield:** 2 servings

🕐 **Prep time:** 10 minutes

🍞 **Cook time:** 20 minutes

NUTRITIONAL INFORMATION (PER SERVING)

- ❖ Calories: 500
- ❖ Fat: 40g
- ❖ Protein: 30g
- ❖ Net Carbs: 4g
- ❖ Fiber: 1g

TIPS

- ❖ *Let the juiciest pork chops rest for a few minutes after cooking before serving. This allows the juices to redistribute throughout the meat.*

- ❖ *If you have fresh herbs on hand, consider adding chopped thyme or rosemary to the mushroom sauce for an extra layer of flavor.*

INGREDIENTS

- ☐ *2 pork chops*
- ☐ *1 cup mushrooms, sliced*
- ☐ *1/2 cup heavy cream*
- ☐ *2 tablespoons butter*
- ☐ *1 clove garlic, minced*
- ☐ *Salt and pepper to taste*
- ☐ *Fresh thyme for garnish*

INSTRUCTIONS

1. Season the pork chops with salt and pepper.

2. Heat a skillet over medium heat and add 1 tablespoon of butter. Add the pork chops and cook for 4-5 minutes on each side until golden brown is cooked through. Remove from the skillet and set aside.

3. In the same skillet, add the remaining butter and garlic. Cook until fragrant, about 1 minute.

4. Add the mushrooms and cook until they are softened about 5 minutes.

5. Pour in the heavy cream and bring to a simmer. Cook for 2-3 minutes or until the sauce thickens.

6. Return the pork chops to the skillet and coat them with the creamy mushroom sauce.

7. Garnish with fresh thyme and serve.

Keto Creamy Garlic Chicken

🍽 **Yield:** 2 servings

🕐 **Prep time:** 10 minutes

🍞 **Cook time:** 20 minutes

NUTRITIONAL INFORMATION (PER SERVING)

* Calories: 400
* Fat: 28g
* Protein: 35g
* Net Carbs: 2g
* Fiber: 0g

TIPS

* *Pair the creamy garlic chicken with a cauliflower mash or zucchini noodles for a satisfying keto dinner.*

* *Add a pinch of red pepper flakes to the sauce for a bit of heat.*

INGREDIENTS

- ☐ *2 boneless, skinless chicken breasts*
- ☐ *1 tablespoon olive oil*
- ☐ *1/2 cup heavy cream*
- ☐ *2 cloves garlic, minced*
- ☐ *1/4 cup grated Parmesan cheese*
- ☐ *Salt and pepper to taste*
- ☐ *Fresh thyme or parsley, chopped for garnish*

INSTRUCTIONS

1. Season the chicken breasts with salt and pepper.

2. Heat the olive oil in a skillet over medium heat. Add the chicken and cook until golden brown on both sides, about 5-7 minutes per side. Remove the chicken from the skillet and set aside.

3. In the same skillet, add the minced garlic and cook until fragrant, about 1 minute.

4. Stir in the heavy cream and Parmesan cheese. Simmer for a few minutes until the sauce thickens.

5. Return the chicken to the skillet and coat it with the creamy garlic sauce.

6. Garnish with fresh thyme or parsley and serve.

Keto Eggplant Parmesan

🍽 **Yield:** 2 servings

🕐 **Prep time:** 15 minutes

🍞 **Cook time:** 25 minutes

NUTRITIONAL INFORMATION (PER SERVING)

* Calories: 400
* Fat: 30g
* Protein: 20g
* Net Carbs: 10g
* Fiber: 5g

TIPS

* *To save time, use pre-made cauliflower rice, which is available in the frozen section of most grocery stores.*

* *Add chopped nuts like almonds or cashews for added crunch and texture.*

* *Add cooked shrimp or diced chicken breast to the fried rice to increase the protein content.*

* *Spice it up with a dash of chili flakes or a splash of hot sauce for an extra kick of flavor.*

INGREDIENTS

- [ ] *1 medium eggplant, sliced into 1/2-inch rounds*
- [ ] *1 cup marinara sauce (keto-friendly)*
- [ ] *1 cup shredded mozzarella cheese*
- [ ] *1/4 cup grated Parmesan cheese*
- [ ] *1/4 cup almond flour*
- [ ] *1 egg, beaten*
- [ ] *2 tablespoons olive oil*
- [ ] *Salt and pepper to taste*
- [ ] *Fresh basil for garnish*

INSTRUCTIONS

1. Preheat the oven to 400°F (200°C).

2. Season the eggplant slices with salt and pepper. Dip each slice in the beaten egg, then coat with almond flour.

3. Heat olive oil in a skillet over medium heat. Add the eggplant slices and cook for 2-3 minutes on each side or until golden brown. Remove from the skillet and set aside.

4. In a baking dish, spread a layer of marinara sauce. Place the eggplant slices on top of the sauce, then cover with more marinara sauce.

5. Sprinkle the shredded mozzarella and grated Parmesan cheese over the eggplant.

6. Bake in the oven for 15-20 minutes or until the cheese is melted and bubbly.

7. Garnish with fresh basil and serve.

Keto Zucchini Lasagna

🍽️ **Yield:** 2 servings

🕐 **Prep time:** 20 minutes

🍞 **Cook time:** 40 minutes

NUTRITIONAL INFORMATION (PER SERVING)

- ❖ Calories: 450
- ❖ Fat: 30g
- ❖ Protein: 35g
- ❖ Net Carbs: 8g
- ❖ Fiber: 2g

TIPS

- ❖ *To prevent the lasagna from being too watery, grill or bake the zucchini slices for a few minutes before assembling the lasagna to remove excess moisture.*

- ❖ *Let the lasagna rest for 10-15 minutes after baking to allow it to set and make it easier to slice and serve.*

INGREDIENTS

- [ ] *2 large zucchinis, sliced lengthwise into thin strips*
- [ ] *1/2 lb ground beef*
- [ ] *1 cup marinara sauce (keto-friendly)*
- [ ] *1 cup ricotta cheese*
- [ ] *1/2 cup shredded mozzarella cheese*
- [ ] *1/4 cup grated Parmesan cheese*
- [ ] *1 egg*
- [ ] *2 cloves garlic, minced*
- [ ] *Salt and pepper to taste*
- [ ] *Fresh basil for garnish*

INSTRUCTIONS

1. Preheat the oven to 375°F (190°C).

2. In a skillet, cook the ground beef and garlic over medium heat until the meat is browned. Drain any excess fat.

3. Stir in the marinara sauce and simmer for 5 minutes—season with salt and pepper to taste.

4. Mix the ricotta cheese, egg, and a pinch of salt and pepper in a bowl.

5. Layer the zucchini strips, ricotta mixture, meat sauce, and mozzarella cheese in a baking dish. Repeat the layers until all ingredients are used, ending with a layer of mozzarella and Parmesan cheese on top.

6. Cover with foil and bake for 30 minutes. Remove the foil and bake for 10 minutes or until the cheese is melted and bubbly.

7. Let the lasagna rest for 10 minutes before serving. Garnish with fresh basil.

SNACKS AND DESSERTS: GUILT-FREE TREATS

Keto Mini Cheesecake Bites

🍴 **Yield:** 12 bites

🕐 **Prep time:** 15 minutes

🍞 **Cook time:** 18 minutes

NUTRITIONAL INFORMATION (PER BITE)

- ❖ Calories: 120
- ❖ Fat: 10g
- ❖ Protein: 3g
- ❖ Net Carbs: 2g
- ❖ Fiber: 0.5g

INGREDIENTS

- ☐ *8 oz cream cheese, softened*
- ☐ *1/4 cup erythritol or sweetener of choice*
- ☐ *1 egg*
- ☐ *1/2 teaspoon vanilla extract*
- ☐ *1/2 cup almond flour (for crust)*
- ☐ *2 tablespoons butter, melted (for crust)*
- ☐ *1 tablespoon erythritol or sweetener of choice (for crust)*

INSTRUCTIONS

1. Preheat the oven to 350°F (175°C) and line a mini muffin pan with paper liners.

2. For the crust, combine the almond flour, melted butter, and erythritol in a mixing bowl. Mix until well combined.

3. Press about a teaspoon of the crust mixture into the bottom of each muffin liner.

4. In another mixing bowl, beat the cream cheese, erythritol, egg, and vanilla extract until smooth and creamy.

5. Spoon the cheesecake filling over the crust in each muffin liner, filling them almost to the top.

6. Bake for 15-18 minutes or until the cheesecakes are set.

7. Allow the cheesecake bites to cool in the pan for a few minutes before transferring them to the refrigerator to chill for at least 2 hours.

8. Serve chilled, and enjoy!

Keto Chocolate Chip Cookies

🍽 **Yield:** 12 cookies

🕐 **Prep time:** 10 minutes

🍞 **Cook time:** 12 minutes

NUTRITIONAL INFORMATION (PER COOKIE)

- ❖ Calories: 140
- ❖ Fat: 12g
- ❖ Protein: 3g
- ❖ Net Carbs: 2g
- ❖ Fiber: 2g

TIPS

- ❖ *For added crunch, mix in some chopped nuts like pecans or walnuts.*

- ❖ *If you prefer softer cookies, reduce the baking time by a couple of minutes.*

- ❖ *Store the cookies in an airtight container at room temperature for up to a week, or freeze them for more extended storage.*

INGREDIENTS

- ☐ *1 1/2 cups almond flour*
- ☐ *1/4 cup coconut oil, melted*
- ☐ *1/4 cup erythritol or sweetener of choice*
- ☐ *1 large egg*
- ☐ *1 teaspoon vanilla extract*
- ☐ *1/2 teaspoon baking powder*
- ☐ *1/4 teaspoon salt*
- ☐ *1/3 cup sugar-free chocolate chips*

INSTRUCTIONS

1. Preheat the oven to 350°F (175°C) and line a baking sheet with parchment paper.

2. Combine the almond flour, erythritol, baking powder, and salt in a mixing bowl.

3. Add the melted coconut oil, egg, and vanilla extract to the dry ingredients. Mix until well combined.

4. Fold in the sugar-free chocolate chips.

5. Scoop out tablespoon-sized portions of the dough and place them on the prepared baking sheet, flattening them slightly.

6. Bake for 10-12 minutes or until the edges are golden brown.

7. Allow the cookies to cool on the baking sheet for a few minutes before transferring them to a wire rack to cool completely.

Keto Lemon Bars

🍽 **Yield:** 9 bars

🕐 **Prep time:** 10 minutes

🎩 **Cook time:** 25 minutes

NUTRITIONAL INFORMATION (PER BAR)

- ❖ Calories: 150
- ❖ Fat: 12g
- ❖ Protein: 5g
- ❖ Net Carbs: 3g
- ❖ Fiber: 2g

INGREDIENTS

For the crust:

- ☐ *1 cup almond flour*
- ☐ *1/4 cup unsalted butter, melted*
- ☐ *2 tablespoons erythritol*
- ☐ *1/2 teaspoon vanilla extract*

For the filling:

- ☐ *3 large eggs*
- ☐ *1/2 cup erythritol*
- ☐ *1/2 cup lemon juice*
- ☐ *2 tablespoons lemon zest*
- ☐ *1/4 cup almond flour*

INSTRUCTIONS

1. Preheat the oven to 350°F (175°C) and line an 8x8-inch baking dish with parchment paper.

2. Combine the almond flour, melted butter, erythritol, and vanilla extract for the crust in a mixing bowl. Press the mixture into the bottom of the prepared baking dish.

3. Bake the crust for 10 minutes, then remove from the oven.

4. In another mixing bowl, whisk together the eggs, erythritol, lemon juice, and zest for the filling. Gradually whisk in the almond flour.

5. Pour the filling over the baked crust and return to the oven.

6. Bake for 15-18 minutes or until the filling is set.

7. Let the lemon bars cool completely before slicing and serving.

Keto Raspberry Swirl Cheesecake

🍽️ **Yield:** 8 servings

🕐 **Prep time:** 15 minutes

🍞 **Cook time:** 45 minutes

NUTRITIONAL INFORMATION (PER SERVING)

- Calories: 320
- Fat: 28g
- Protein: 7g
- Net Carbs: 5g
- Fiber: 2g

INGREDIENTS

For the filling:

- ☐ *16 oz cream cheese, softened*
- ☐ *1/2 cup erythritol*
- ☐ *2 large eggs*
- ☐ *1 teaspoon vanilla extract*

For the crust:

- ☐ *1 cup almond flour*
- ☐ *1/4 cup unsalted butter, melted*
- ☐ *1 tablespoon erythritol*

For the raspberry swirl:

- ☐ *1/2 cup raspberries*
- ☐ *1 tablespoon erythritol*

INSTRUCTIONS

1. Preheat the oven to 325°F (160°C) and line a 9-inch springform pan with parchment paper.

2. Combine the almond flour, melted butter, and erythritol in a bowl for the crust. Press the mixture into the bottom of the prepared pan.

3. Bake the crust for 10 minutes, then remove from the oven and let cool.

4. For the filling, beat the cream cheese and erythritol until smooth. Add the eggs one at a time, beating well after each addition. Stir in the vanilla extract.

5. Pour the filling over the cooled crust.

6. For the raspberry swirl, blend the raspberries and erythritol in a blender or food processor until smooth. Drop spoonfuls of the raspberry mixture onto the cheesecake filling and use a toothpick to swirl it into the filling.

7. Bake the cheesecake for 35-40 minutes, or until the edges are set but the center is still slightly jiggly.

8. Turn off the oven and leave the cheesecake inside with the door closed for an additional hour.

9. Remove the cheesecake from the oven and let it cool to room temperature, then refrigerate for at least 4 hours or overnight before serving.

Keto Chocolate Peanut Butter Fat Bombs

🍽️ **Yield:** 12 fat bombs

🕐 **Prep time:** 10 minutes

🍞 **Cook time:** 0 minutes (plus chilling time)

NUTRITIONAL INFORMATION (PER FAT BOMB)

- ❖ Calories: 120
- ❖ Fat: 11g
- ❖ Protein: 2g
- ❖ Net Carbs: 2g
- ❖ Fiber: 1g

INGREDIENTS

- ☐ *1/2 cup natural peanut butter (no added sugar)*
- ☐ *1/4 cup coconut oil*
- ☐ *1/4 cup unsweetened cocoa powder*
- ☐ *2 tablespoons erythritol or sweetener of choice*
- ☐ *1/2 teaspoon vanilla extract*
- ☐ *A pinch of salt*

INSTRUCTIONS

1. Combine the peanut butter and coconut oil in a microwave-safe bowl. Microwave for 30 seconds or until melted and smooth.

2. Stir in the cocoa powder, erythritol, vanilla extract, and salt until well combined.

3. Pour the mixture into silicone molds or mini muffin liners.

4. Place in the freezer for at least 1 hour or until the fat bombs are solid.

5. Once set, remove the fat bombs from the molds and store them in an airtight container in the refrigerator or freezer.

Keto Almond Joy Bars

🍴 **Yield:** 8 bars

🕐 **Prep time:** 15 minutes

🎩 **Cook time:** 0 minutes (plus chilling time)

NUTRITIONAL INFORMATION (PER BAR)

- ❖ Calories: 180
- ❖ Fat: 16g
- ❖ Protein: 2g
- ❖ Net Carbs: 3g
- ❖ Fiber: 3g

INGREDIENTS

- ☐ *1 cup unsweetened shredded coconut*
- ☐ *1/3 cup coconut cream*
- ☐ *2 tablespoons erythritol or sweetener of choice*
- ☐ *1/2 teaspoon vanilla extract*
- ☐ *16 whole almonds*
- ☐ *1/2 cup sugar-free dark chocolate chips*
- ☐ *1 tablespoon coconut oil*

INSTRUCTIONS

1. Combine the shredded coconut, coconut cream, erythritol, and vanilla extract in a mixing bowl. Mix until well combined.

2. Press the mixture into a lined 8x4-inch loaf pan, creating an even layer.

3. Press two almonds into each bar, evenly spacing them along the length of the pan.

4. Freeze the coconut mixture for about 30 minutes or until firm.

5. In a microwave-safe bowl, melt the dark chocolate chips and coconut oil together, stirring until smooth.

6. Remove the coconut mixture from the freezer and cut it into 8 bars.

7. Dip each bar into the melted chocolate, ensuring it's fully coated. Place the coated bars on a parchment-lined tray.

8. Refrigerate the bars for about 15 minutes or until the chocolate is set.

9. Store the Keto Almond Joy Bars in the refrigerator until ready to serve.

SOUPS AND SALADS

Keto Creamy Cauliflower Soup

🍽 **Yield:** 4 servings

🕐 **Prep time:** 10 minutes

👨‍🍳 **Cook time:** 25 minutes

NUTRITIONAL INFORMATION (PER SERVING)

* Calories: 250
* Fat: 22g
* Protein: 4g
* Net Carbs: 6g
* Fiber: 3g

TIPS

* *Blend it until completely pureed for a smoother soup. Blend it less or leave some cauliflower pieces whole for a chunkier texture.*

* *Experiment with different cheeses for variations in flavor, such as smoked gouda or pepper jack.*

INGREDIENTS

- [ ] *1 head cauliflower, chopped*
- [ ] *2 tablespoons butter*
- [ ] *1 small onion, diced*
- [ ] *2 cloves garlic, minced*
- [ ] *3 cups chicken broth*
- [ ] *1 cup heavy cream*
- [ ] *Salt and pepper to taste*
- [ ] *Optional toppings: shredded cheddar cheese, crumbled bacon, chopped chives*

INSTRUCTIONS

1. Melt the butter in a large pot over medium heat. Add the onion and garlic and sauté until softened for about 5 minutes.

2. Add the chopped cauliflower and chicken broth. Bring to a boil, then reduce heat and simmer until the cauliflower is tender about 15-20 minutes.

3. Use an immersion blender to puree the soup until smooth. Stir in the heavy cream and season with salt and pepper.

4. Serve hot, garnished with optional toppings if desired.

Keto Avocado Chicken Salad

🍽 **Yield:** 2 servings

🕐 **Prep time:** 15 minutes

🍞 **Cook time:** 0 minutes

NUTRITIONAL INFORMATION (PER SERVING)

- ❖ Calories: 400
- ❖ Fat: 30g
- ❖ Protein: 25g
- ❖ Net Carbs: 4g
- ❖ Fiber: 5g

TIPS

- ❖ *Use rotisserie chicken for a quick and convenient option.*
- ❖ *Add diced bell peppers or sliced almonds to the salad for extra crunch.*

INGREDIENTS

- ☐ *2 cups cooked chicken, shredded*
- ☐ *1 large avocado, diced*
- ☐ *1/4 cup mayonnaise (keto-friendly)*
- ☐ *2 tablespoons cilantro, chopped*
- ☐ *1 tablespoon lime juice*
- ☐ *Salt and pepper to taste*
- ☐ *Optional: diced red onion, diced cucumber*

INSTRUCTIONS

1. Combine the shredded chicken, diced avocado, mayonnaise, cilantro, and lime juice in a mixing bowl. Mix until well combined.

2. Season with salt and pepper to taste. Add optional ingredients if desired.

3. Serve immediately or chill in the refrigerator until ready to eat.

Keto Zucchini Noodle Salad with Pesto

🍽 **Yield:** 2 servings

🕐 **Prep time:** 10 minutes

🍞 **Cook time:** 0 minutes

NUTRITIONAL INFORMATION (PER SERVING)

- ❖ Calories: 200
- ❖ Fat: 16g
- ❖ Protein: 4g
- ❖ Net Carbs: 6g
- ❖ Fiber: 2g

TIPS

- ❖ *If you don't have a spiralizer, use a vegetable peeler to create thin zucchini ribbons.*

- ❖ *For a protein boost, add grilled chicken or shrimp to the salad.*

INGREDIENTS

- [ ] *2 medium zucchinis, spiralized*
- [ ] *1/4 cup pesto (keto-friendly)*
- [ ] *1/4 cup cherry tomatoes, halved*
- [ ] *2 tablespoons pine nuts, toasted*
- [ ] *Salt and pepper to taste*
- [ ] *Optional: shaved Parmesan cheese*

INSTRUCTIONS

1. In a mixing bowl, combine the spiralized zucchini and pesto. Toss until the zucchini noodles are well coated.

2. Add the cherry tomatoes and pine nuts. Toss gently.

3. Season with salt and pepper to taste. Add optional shaved Parmesan cheese if desired.

4. Serve immediately or chill in the refrigerator for a refreshing salad.

Keto Broccoli Cheddar Soup

🍽 **Yield:** 4 servings

🕐 **Prep time:** 10 minutes

🍞 **Cook time:** 20 minutes

NUTRITIONAL INFORMATION (PER SERVING)

* Calories: 350
* Fat: 30g
* Protein: 12g
* Net Carbs: 6g
* Fiber: 2g

TIPS

* *Add an extra 1/2 cup of cheese or a few ounces of cream cheese for a thicker soup.*

* *Garnish with extra shredded cheddar and crispy bacon bits for added flavor and texture.*

INGREDIENTS

- ☐ *4 cups broccoli florets*
- ☐ *2 cups chicken broth*
- ☐ *1 cup heavy cream*
- ☐ *1 1/2 cups shredded cheddar cheese*
- ☐ *1/4 cup diced onion*
- ☐ *2 cloves garlic, minced*
- ☐ *2 tablespoons butter*
- ☐ *Salt and pepper to taste*

INSTRUCTIONS

1. Melt the butter in a large pot over medium heat. Add the onion and garlic, and sauté until softened, about 5 minutes.

2. Add the broccoli florets and chicken broth. Bring to a boil, then reduce heat and simmer until the broccoli is tender, about 10 minutes.

3. Use an immersion blender to slightly puree the soup, leaving some broccoli chunks for texture.

4. Stir in the heavy cream and shredded cheddar cheese. Cook until the cheese is melted and the soup is heated through.

5. Season with salt and pepper to taste. Serve hot.

Keto Greek Salad

🍽 **Yield:** 2 servings

🕐 **Prep time:** 10 minutes

🍞 **Cook time:** 0 minutes

NUTRITIONAL INFORMATION (PER SERVING)

- ❖ Calories: 250
- ❖ Fat: 22g
- ❖ Protein: 5g
- ❖ Net Carbs: 5g
- ❖ Fiber: 2g

TIPS

- *Use Greek feta cheese made from sheep's milk for a more authentic flavor.*
- *Add grilled chicken, steak, or shrimp to make it a filling main dish.*

INGREDIENTS

- ☐ *2 cups romaine lettuce, chopped*
- ☐ *1/2 cup cherry tomatoes, halved*
- ☐ *1/4 cup cucumber, sliced*
- ☐ *1/4 cup Kalamata olives, pitted*
- ☐ *1/4 cup feta cheese, crumbled*
- ☐ *2 tablespoons olive oil*
- ☐ *1 tablespoon red wine vinegar*
- ☐ *1/2 teaspoon dried oregano*
- ☐ *Salt and pepper to taste*

INSTRUCTIONS

1. Combine the romaine lettuce, cherry tomatoes, cucumber, Kalamata olives, and feta cheese in a large bowl.

2. Whisk together the olive oil, red wine vinegar, dried oregano, salt, and pepper in a small bowl.

3. Pour the dressing over the salad and toss to combine.

4. Serve immediately or chill in the refrigerator until ready to eat.

Keto Tomato Basil Soup

🍽 **Yield:** 4 servings

🕐 **Prep time:** 5 minutes

🍞 **Cook time:** 20 minutes

NUTRITIONAL INFORMATION (PER SERVING)

- ❖ Calories: 180
- ❖ Fat: 16g
- ❖ Protein: 2g
- ❖ Net Carbs: 5g
- ❖ Fiber: 1g

TIPS

- ❖ *Add more heavy cream or blend in some softened cream cheese for a creamier soup.*
- ❖ *Roast the tomatoes and garlic before adding them to the soup for a richer flavor.*

INGREDIENTS

- ☐ *2 cans (14.5 oz each) of diced tomatoes, undrained*
- ☐ *1 cup chicken broth*
- ☐ *1/2 cup heavy cream*
- ☐ *1/4 cup fresh basil, chopped*
- ☐ *2 cloves garlic, minced*
- ☐ *2 tablespoons olive oil*
- ☐ *Salt and pepper to taste*

INSTRUCTIONS

1. In a large pot, heat the olive oil over medium heat. Add the minced garlic and cook until fragrant, about 1 minute.

2. Add the diced tomatoes (with their juice) and chicken broth. Bring to a simmer and cook for 15 minutes.

3. Use an immersion blender to puree the soup until smooth.

4. Stir in the heavy cream and chopped basil. Season with salt and pepper to taste.

5. Cook for an additional 2-3 minutes or until heated through. Serve hot.

CHAPTERS 10:
90-DAY KETO MEAL PLAN FOR SENIORS

Week 1-4: Introduction to Keto for Seniors

Focus: Simple and easy-to-prepare meals to ease into the keto lifestyle.

DAY	BREAKFAST	LUNCH	DINNER
1	Keto Egg Muffins	Keto Greek Salad	Keto Lemon Herb Roasted Chicken Thighs
2	Keto Avocado Toast	Keto Creamy Cauliflower Soup	Keto Beef Stir-Fry with Broccoli
3	Keto Berry Smoothie	Keto Zucchini Noodle Salad with Pesto	Keto Pork Chops with Creamy Mushroom Sauce
4	Keto Chia Seed Pudding	Keto Avocado Chicken Salad	Keto Lemon Garlic Butter Salmon
5	Keto BLT Lettuce Wrap	Keto Broccoli Cheddar Soup	Keto Chicken Caesar Lettuce Wraps
6	Keto Chocolate Avocado Mousse	Keto Tuna Salad Stuffed Avocados	Keto Zucchini Lasagna
7	Keto Almond Butter Energy Balls	Keto Tomato Basil Soup	Keto Cajun Shrimp and Sausage Skillet

Repeat similar patterns for the remaining weeks in this phase, experimenting with different combinations of the recipes provided.

Week 5-8: Building Confidence in Keto Cooking

Focus: Incorporating various ingredients and exploring new flavors while keeping meals simple.

- Introduce one new recipe per day while repeating familiar ones to build confidence.

- Experiment with different herbs and spices to enhance flavors.

- Focus on meal prep techniques like batch cooking and storing leftovers for convenience.

DAY	BREAKFAST	LUNCH	DINNER
1	Keto Almond Butter Energy Balls	Keto Greek Salad with Grilled Chicken	Keto Creamy Garlic Chicken
2	Keto Chocolate Avocado Mousse	Keto Tuna Stuffed Bell Peppers	Keto Beef and Mushroom Stroganoff
3	Keto Peanut Butter Cookies	Keto Chicken Caesar Salad	Keto Lemon Herb Roasted Chicken
4	Keto Berry Smoothie	Keto Cheesy Cauliflower Bites	Keto Pork Chops with Creamy Mushroom Sauce
5	Keto Chia Seed Pudding	Keto Zucchini Noodle Salad with Pesto	Keto Shrimp and Avocado Salad

6	Keto BLT Lettuce Wrap	Keto Avocado Chicken Salad	Keto Chicken Avocado Salad
7	Keto Egg Muffins	Keto Tomato Basil Soup	Keto Cajun Shrimp and Sausage Skillet

Week 9-12: Diversifying Your Keto Meals

Focus: Expand your meal repertoire and try more diverse and complex recipes.

❖ Start incorporating more seafood and vegetarian options into your meals.

❖ Experiment with keto-friendly international cuisines, such as Mediterranean or Asian-inspired dishes.

❖ Try making keto versions of traditional favorites, like cauliflower crust pizza or zucchini noodle pasta.

DAY	BREAKFAST	LUNCH	DINNER
1	Keto Chocolate Peanut Butter Fat Bombs	Keto Creamy Cauliflower Soup	Keto Zucchini Lasagna
2	Keto Almond Joy Bars	Keto Broccoli Cheddar Soup	Keto Beef Stir-Fry with Broccoli
3	Keto Peanut Butter Cookies	Keto Greek Salad	Keto Lemon Garlic Butter Salmon

4	Keto Berry Smoothie	Keto Avocado Chicken Salad	Keto Creamy Garlic Chicken
5	Keto Chia Seed Pudding	Keto Zucchini Noodle Salad with Pesto	Keto Beef and Mushroom Stroganoff
6	Keto BLT Lettuce Wrap	Keto Chicken Caesar Salad	Keto Lemon Herb Roasted Chicken
7	Keto Egg Muffins	Keto Tomato Basil Soup	Keto Pork Chops with Creamy Mushroom Sauce

Week 13-16: Mastering Keto Meal Planning

Focus: Developing a routine for planning and preparing meals in advance to make the keto lifestyle sustainable.

- Plan your meals for the week ahead, including snacks and desserts.

- Focus on using seasonal and fresh ingredients for variety and nutrition.

- Practice making larger batches of meals to freeze and reheat later.

DAY	BREAKFAST	LUNCH	DINNER
1	Keto Almond Butter Energy Balls	Keto Greek Salad with Grilled Chicken	Keto Shrimp and Avocado Salad
2	Keto Chocolate Avocado Mousse	Keto Tuna Stuffed Bell Peppers	Keto Chicken Avocado Salad
3	Keto Peanut Butter Cookies	Keto Cheesy Cauliflower Bites	Keto Zucchini Lasagna

4	Keto Berry Smoothie	Keto Chicken Caesar Salad	Keto Creamy Garlic Chicken
5	Keto Chia Seed Pudding	Keto Zucchini Noodle Salad with Pesto	Keto Beef Stir-Fry with Broccoli
6	Keto BLT Lettuce Wrap	Keto Avocado Chicken Salad	Keto Lemon Herb Roasted Chicken
7	Keto Egg Muffins	Keto Tomato Basil Soup	Keto Cajun Shrimp and Sausage Skillet

Tips for Adapting Meals to Your Preferences

❖ Customize recipes based on your dietary needs and preferences, such as substituting ingredients or adjusting portion sizes.

❖ Pay attention to how your body responds to different foods and adjust your meal plan accordingly.

❖ Stay hydrated and complement your meals with keto-friendly beverages like water infused with lemon or herbal teas.

This meal plan is a guide to help you transition into and maintain a keto lifestyle. Feel free to adjust the recipes and meal combinations to suit your tastes and nutritional needs.

Conversion Tables

Flour

1 cup	125 grams
¾ cup	94 grams
2/3 cup	83 grams
½ cup	63 grams
1/3 cup	42 grams
1/4 cup	31 grams
1 tablespoon	8 grams
1 teaspoon	3 grams

Oil

1 ½ cup	12 fl oz	24 tbsp	72 tsp
1 cup	8 fl oz	16 tbsp	48 tsp
¾ cup	6 fl oz	12 tbsp	36 tsp
2/3 cup	5.33 fl oz	10.5 tbsp	32 tsp
½ cup	4 fl oz	8 tbsp	24 tsp
1/3 cup	2.67 fl oz	5.33 tbsp	16 tsp
¼ cup	2 fl oz	4 tbsp	12 tsp
1 tablespoon	0.5 fl oz	15 ml	14 g

Water

2 cups	16 fl oz	473.18 ml
1 ½ cups	12 fl oz	354.88 ml
1 cup	8 fl oz	236.59 ml
3/4 cup	6 fl oz	177.44 ml
2/3 cup	5.33 fl oz	157.73 ml
1/2 cup	4 fl oz	118.29 ml
1/3 cup	2.67 fl oz	78.86 ml
1/4 cup	2 fl oz	59.15 ml

Milk

1 cup	8 fl oz	240 ml
3/4 cup	6 fl oz	180 ml
2/3 cup	5.3 fl oz	160 ml
1/2 cup	4 fl oz	120 ml
1/3 cup	2.7 fl oz	80 ml
1/4 cup	2 fl oz	60 ml
1 tablespoon	0.5 fl oz	15 ml
1 teaspoon	0.17 fl oz	5 ml

Yeast

1 pocket (1/4 oz)	2 ¼ teaspoons, 7 grams
1 teaspoon	3.1 grams
1 tablespoon	9.3 grams

- To substitute active dry for instant yeast, increase the yeast amount by 25%.
- To substitute instant yeast for active dry, decrease the required amount of yeast by 25%

Sugar (granulated)

1 ½ cup	300 grams	24 tbsp	72 tsp
1 cup	200 grams	16 tbsp	48 tsp
¾ cup	150 grams	12 tbsp	36 tsp
2/3 cup	134 grams	10.5 tbsp	32 tsp
½ cup	100 grams	8 tbsp	24 tsp
1/3 cup	67 grams	5.33 tbsp	16 tsp
¼ cup	50 grams	4 tbsp	12 tsp
1 tablespoon	12.5 grams		

Sugar (powdered)

1 ½ cup	180 grams	24 tbsp	72 tsp
1 cup	120 grams	16 tbsp	48 tsp
¾ cup	90 grams	12 tbsp	36 tsp
2/3 cup	80 grams	10.5 tbsp	32 tsp
½ cup	60 grams	8 tbsp	24 tsp
1/3 cup	40 grams	5.33 tbsp	16 tsp
¼ cup	30 grams	4 tbsp	12 tsp
1 tablespoon	8 grams		

Butter

1 cup	2 sticks	8 oz	226 g
¾ cup	1 ½ sticks	6 oz	170 g
2/3 cup	1 1/3 sticks	5.33 oz	151 g
½ cup	1 stick	4 oz	113 g
1/3 cup	0.67 stick	2.67 oz	75 g
¼ cup	0.50 stick	2 oz	56.7 g
1 tablespoon		0.5 oz	14.2 g
1 tablespoon		0.17 oz	4.7 g

Made in the USA
Columbia, SC
28 September 2024